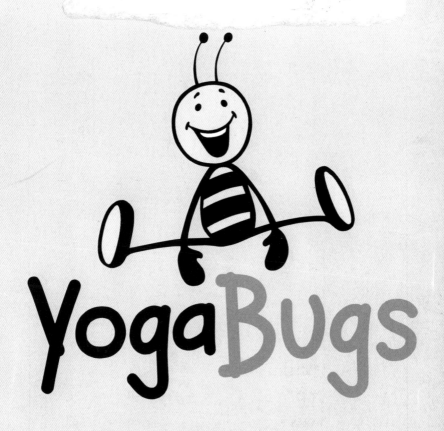

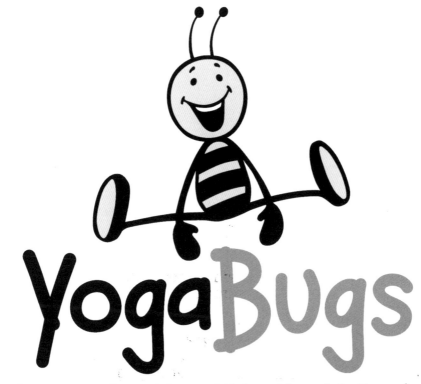

YogaBugs

The One Bug Your Kids Should Catch

Fenella Lindsell

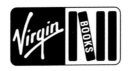

I would like to dedicate this book to my husband Rob and to my family, George, Felix, Barney and Letty, and to YogaBugs past, present and future.

First published in Great Britain in 2008 by
Virgin Books Ltd
Thames Wharf Studios
Rainville Road
London
W6 9HA

A catalogue record for this book is available from the British Library.

ISBN 978 0 7535 1336 1

The paper used in this book is a natural, recyclable product made from wood grown in sustainable forests. The manufacturing process conforms to the regulations of the country of origin.

Design by Virgin Books

Printed and bound by Butler & Tanner

YogaBugs character illustrations by Barking Dog Art. Photographs © YogaBugs. All other illustrations © Virgin Books

Contents

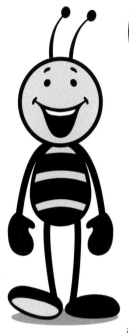

Introduction
Who Are YogaBugs?

I am writing this book in the hope that sharing my experience and that of the YogaBugs I have taught over the years will inspire and encourage you to set out on your own yoga journey, together with your children. All you need is an open mind, a warm heart and plenty of energy!

YogaBugs is aimed at 2½–7-year-olds, an age group whose imagination is limitless: they are flexible, enthusiastic and full of energy. You are simply trying to develop and harness all these wonderful gifts for the future. Currently YogaBugs is taught as a class through a network of teachers in nurseries, schools, health clubs and community centres throughout the UK and Ireland. This book gives you the chance to join in and share your child's enjoyment, interest, excitement and the benefit they will gain from the adventures and games.

YogaBugs turns yoga, an activity traditionally associated with adults, into a fun, creative playground for children through a series of stories, journeys and games that will help them at many different levels.

Before we set off on our own adventure, I want to tell you what you will discover as we travel through this book together. We'll begin with the positive benefits of yoga to your child – and, believe me, there are many, for both their physical and mental health.

The next part of the book puts theory into practice with breathing and warm-up techniques. Next come the YogaBugs adventures – the central part of this book – which include suggestions to help the children relax, enjoy visualisation techniques and, finally, benefit from the positive affirmations contained in the stories.

After this you'll find detailed information about the warm-up and breathing exercises as well as the instructions on the best way postures can be done to gain most benefit. And, for those of you who are interested, I've included a bit about the history of YogaBugs and how it all came about.

I hope you and your children have as much fun carrying out all the activities in this book as I have had writing them!

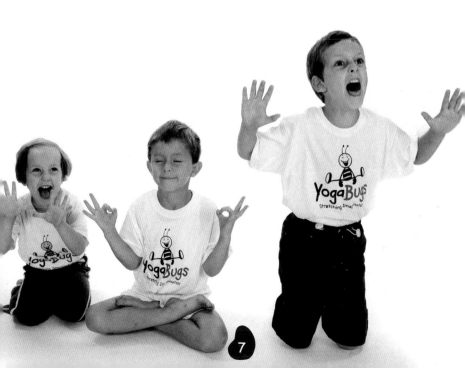

Chapter 1
Why We Should All Catch the Bug!

From my own practice, I can say that teaching YogaBugs is thrilling and totally absorbing. Capturing a child's imagination through a creative and magical story is so uplifting. Children have no idea about personal space; they press towards you in their enthusiasm to be involved. They spill out excited ideas that might be about their new dress, toy car, Sam's pirate party on Saturday or just the sheer joy of the moment. This connection with a child is so special. There are few physical activities that small children actually do better than grown-ups, but yoga is certainly one of them. They are flexible and energetic, and have boundless imaginations!

YogaBugs is creative, imaginative and fun! Yoga postures, breathing and relaxation techniques are woven together into wild adventures and heroic journeys. Children fly on magic carpets, travel on mystical birds, ride on dolphins, take space rockets to the moon and dance in underwater palaces. Yoga with children is as limitless as your imagination.

The breathing and warm-up techniques help children to focus; the posture work strengthens and tones their bodies; relaxation and visualisation techniques help their concentration and improve their sleep patterns. Stories are as much fun for adults as for children and provide an enchanting experience! YogaBugs need no incentive to become superheroes, scary snakes or wicked pirates – their imagination kicks in and you can be there to enjoy it with them. Sharing yoga with children transcends the boundaries of age and physical ability.

Yoga also helps children to become aware of and respect the needs and feelings of others. They learn to follow rules while making and expressing choices, plans and decisions. Through yoga children can be taught to play co-operatively, take turns and share resources. Stories are also helpful for children with additional needs, and, in the safe environment of a class – one to one or as a small group – these children can really show improvements. (See the section on additional needs on Page 172).

Many headteachers, class teachers, and teaching assistants have re-marked on the beneficial effects YogaBugs has had on their children. Richard Dell, who was headmaster at Newton Preparatory School in Battersea, London (which was one of the first to start YogaBugs in 1997), said that the results were impressive.

'Yoga works at a different level,' he said, 'teaching the children to link body and mind in a language they can understand. It's challenging but contemplative and I'm convinced it helps children focus better on their schoolwork. Life in London moves at such a fast pace for young children. This can help them relax and enjoy something peaceful. In my view, it would be wonderful to have it included in the National Curriculum.'

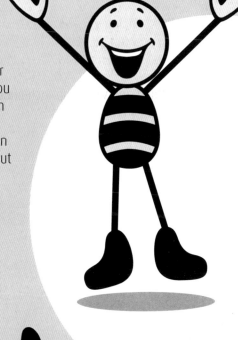

Whatever it is that has brought this book to you, enjoy it, share it with your child or children and remember that, through yoga, together you are helping the next generation to stretch their imaginations, enrich their lives and provide an environment for them to live out their dreams.

Chapter 2
How YogaBugs can Help Your Child

Yoga lays the foundations for a lifelong journey of discovery, familiarity and stability. A child can start yoga at any age. They may imitate parents or siblings from as early as twelve to eighteen months, though they do not become aware of how to control their bodily movements until about two years onwards. What is fundamental is that they have begun a form of exercise and relaxation they will enjoy throughout their lives.

In this modern-day environment children lead a more sedentary lifestyle. There is less emphasis on physical education in schools and more on literacy and numeracy in order to meet the ever-demanding educational targets. Children are being denied their natural freedom of movement, imagination and inherent creativity. Added to this, long hours of television and computer games have led to postural problems and inertia, and – not surprisingly – childhood obesity has become a serious issue. One in four children in England is now obese, according to government statistics.

Yoga is a great way of introducing some much-needed physical activity into your children's daily routine, in a way that they will find enjoyable and fun.

Children practising yoga have no preconceived ideas of what the practice involves. Yoga to them is simply exercise-driven fun. Back arches, twists, forward bends, standing postures and inversions are woven into thrilling stories that capture their imagination.

YOGABUGS – THE KEY BENEFITS

Physical

* Breathing exercises improve concentration, strengthen the abdominal muscles and balance energy levels.

* Postures help support the immune, respiratory, circulatory and digestive systems while strengthening the core stabilising muscles of the abdomen and back.

* Posture work helps to tone the body, maintain joint mobility and develop good posture. It helps children become conscious of their bodies, know how to look after themselves and be more aware of what they eat.

Yoga maintains a child's natural flexibility, which can begin to change from a surprisingly young age, especially once they spend more time at their school desks as opposed to taking part in free-range play, and become distracted by computer games and television.

Boys tend to get stiff in the backs of their legs, which makes touching their toes more of a challenge. In the long term, this lack of flexibility can cause discomfort in the lower back.

* For girls, yoga helps to develop upper-body strength and stability in the knees and ankles.

* Yoga can improve agility in sport and help prevent injury.

Mental

* Yoga improves self-confidence through teaching children breathing techniques and encouraging them to use their voices.

* Postures are designed to release day-to-day anxieties such as separation issues, bullying, lethargy and feelings of negativity. Children often find it easier to express their emotional state in a physical way.

* Relaxation techniques bring clarity and stillness to the mind, allowing for improved memory retention which helps children learn more easily. We absorb information better when our brainwaves are in a slower pattern. When we limit outside distraction and work on the sound of our breath and relaxing our body, our brain waves will naturally slow down.

* Classes help children to develop their own creativity through stories and adventures. Even Albert Einstein said that his ideas always came to him in visual images, which he then interpreted into mathematical formulae. He has been quoted as identifying that the prime feature of intelligence is the capability of using imagery with the information that we know. This process helps to use the whole brain and facilitates children learning through their senses as well as through a more structured approach.

* The practice of yoga improves co-ordination and balance; it promotes healthy sleeping patterns and allows children to explore their intuitive nature and their spirituality.

Behavioural
From my own experience, I have seen changes in children such as described below in terms of their behaviour, attitude, energy and enthusiasm.

* The disruptive or attention-seeking type is acknowledged by turning their negative behaviour around and praising them for what they are able to do.

* The 'I don't want to do this' child can't resist the temptation of being involved in the story and, even though they may take a moment, they will probably be joining you on your magic carpet or when you encounter the lions.

* The very energetic child is often the one, after a few sessions, who is last to come out of final relaxation because they have become so involved in their own richly colourful visualisation.

* Nervous or anxious children find that the posture work,

vocalisation and breathing help them feel freer and more confident in themselves.

* So often children grumble about sore tummies, headaches or bumps and bruises from playtime. They feel tired and unmotivated. Yoga is the perfect opportunity to leave these grumbles behind by distracting them with a wonderful adventure.

* Children just want time, released from deadlines and given the chance to let what is inside, out!

* Making a special time for your child and doing something that enables them to explore, create and share with you can only be an advantage. I think it is pretty good for us as adults too! We still all have that little child inside us and it does us good to connect with it from time to time and to play.

WARMING UP, BREATHING AND RELAXATION

The warm-up
In this section we are going to learn the value of making your child aware of how helpful it is to warm up the body correctly for the YogaBugs adventures and, in so doing, avoid injury to vulnerable areas such as lower back, knees, hips, necks and shoulders.

Warm-up exercises
It is vital that children are correctly warmed up before they start their YogaBugs story, as this will prepare them for their adventures.

We have always found that it is great fun to relate the warm-ups to the story. We pack suitcases with all our favourite things for each adventure and we make sure that our bodies feel fit and strong before we set off.

Naturally this helps to lay good foundations for children in terms of valuing warm-up postures for their sporting activities in the future as well. We practise breathing techniques to give us energy on our journeys into space or for our underwater adventures. In the same way we introduce stretching postures to help us to swim and run faster while strengthening exercises will enable us to row our boats better. Jaw and cheek massages are important to enable us to hear and speak well, while eye exercises will teach our eyes to work better and help us always to see where we are going.

Warm-up exercises are also valuable to keep our backs strong and our hips flexible, and to make sure that our necks and shoulders don't get stiff, as grown-ups' shoulders do! We often complete our warm-ups with a fun round of Sun Salutations. These bring all the warmed-up parts of our bodies together so that we are ready to embark on our adventure. We have great fun greeting the sun and this sequence of postures really encourages children to vocalise and share their enjoyment of the activity.

For a complete list of warm-up activities and instructions on how to do them, turn to Page 132.

THE VALUE OF POSTURE WORK

Stories are designed for children to use their imagination with postures, while learning how to breathe correctly and understand how to relax their bodies. There is often an underlying message in the stories about being kind, sympathetic, understanding, or being helpful and friendly. These aspects are re-identified at the end of the adventure during relaxation and visualisation time.

Preschool children have wonderfully supple bodies, but as soon as they start school their flexibility begins to diminish. Once children conform to social conventions, such as sitting for long periods, their spines will lose their natural mobility and their bodies become less flexible. Through yoga they will maintain the natural gifts of childhood.

Many of the stretches help children who suffer from a wide range of problems, such as digestive upsets and stiffness in the joints and muscles. Postures combined with fun-themed adventures are a guaranteed way to engage young children while teaching them valuable exercise, breathing and relaxation techniques.

Choose from our selection of stories and take your children on a special visit to the circus, to the moon, to a shy giant's house or on a magical ocean adventure. Allow your imagination to roam free with your children and listen to their discoveries while being inspired by their enthusiasm and excitement.

NOTE: A child's natural caution coupled with your careful explanations and instructions will protect them from injury.

BREATHING TECHNIQUES

Rather like teaching a child to warm up correctly before doing sport, giving your child techniques to help them to breathe correctly will naturally reflect in other activities that they do in terms of learning, and in their physical and mental development.

There are a wide variety of breathing exercises that are suitable for children. However, children should not be taught to hold their breath, and these exercises should be used to only help children to understand the calming and energising influences of the breath.

It is fun to identify how breathing makes us feel. For example, we can practise Concertina Breath (see Page 130) and this makes us feel warm; while Sithali Breath (see Page 130) has a cooling effect on our body.

Through yoga the goal is to introduce the breathing techniques gradually until the lungs are stronger; and, in general, the aim is to increase lung capacity. Breathing techniques are particularly good after school because that is when children might be tired and lack oxygen to the brain, and this will give them a much-needed lift.

Breathing exercises can also help improve mood and alleviate feelings of lethargy or negativity. Schoolchildren are given little chance to run around in the fresh air and by the afternoon they are weary from being deskbound, in stuffy rooms, absorbing information. Breathing techniques are also particularly beneficial for children who suffer from symptoms of anxiety or have asthma and other related allergies.

Tell your children that a wise yogi once said, 'YogaBugs have all been given a certain number of breaths in their lives, and that we should all measure our lives by the number of breaths we take rather than in the number of years. Obviously the slower and deeper YogaBugs breathe the longer YogaBugs live!'

Yoga is good for encouraging children to breathe correctly, since in our daily lives we tend to use as little as a third of our lungs' capacity. Teaching abdominal breathing improves digestive functions and tones the abdominal muscles. By learning to control their breathing and take deeper breaths, children can improve their whole sense of wellbeing and outlook.

By giving children some basic breathing techniques, you can also help them to deal with some of the issues that they face on a daily basis, such as reading out loud in class, performing in school assembly, singing a solo, taking part in the school play or just in controlling their anger or moments of frustration where deep breathing can be a really great support.

Space breathing (see Page 171) is a very useful tool, which helps children to get to sleep – it stops the busy mind and helps the child to feel calm inside and out.

For a complete list of breathing techniques and how to do them, turn to Page 130.

WHY CHILDREN NEED TO LEARN TO RELAX

In our deadline-driven lives, children have very little time to reflect and daydream.

This in turn limits their creative ability and can often leave them feeling frustrated and moody. We hope that some of the suggestions that are given in the story part of the book, as well as those detailed in this section, will enable children to feel more fulfilled. This will in turn enable them to find a quiet and peaceful place inside themselves, giving them confidence to be calm and settled.

Relaxation and visualisation techniques

Strengthen a child's powers of concentration by enacting a YogaBugs adventure and they will feel calmer and more grounded. Storytelling is a wonderful way to capture a child's imagination and it is an excellent way to teach children to relax by reliving aspects of the adventures, recreating the colours, light, emotions and sensations and helping them to indulge in those feelings.

Relaxation techniques also provide the structure to introduce children to the benefits of meditation. Details of relaxation techniques and guided visualisations are given at the end of each adventure in the story section of the book.

* Encourage your child to lie as still as possible so that their mind can really picture what you are describing to them.

* Ask them to completely relax their toes, feet, legs, hips, back, fingers, hands, arms, shoulders and neck.

* Tell your child to let their body feel really heavy on the floor as you then lead them into the visualisation you create for them.

* Variation in relaxation can be achieved by getting the children into savasana (the corpse pose) and then just to point and flex their toes for two or three minutes. It has a powerful effect on relaxing their limbs.

* Once your child is calm and still, it is perfect to maintain their attention by giving easy but detailed descriptions.

* Use words that describe a sensation such as soft, silky, fluffy.

* Encourage them to take all their thoughts to that place and let go of any other ones that might stop them enjoying the images that you are creating together.

* This is an important time, too, to make children feel good about themselves in terms of identifying helpful and kind things that they may have done in their adventure.

* This is valuable in helping to make children feel more confident and sure of themselves in the competitive environment that surrounds them in life outside.

* If at any time your child is finding it particularly difficult to relax, you can cup their head in your hands or gently rest your hand on their arm or leg to help them to feel calm.

* It is a lovely time to massage your child's feet or gently stroke their forehead. Touch is very powerful and creates a strong bond between adult and child. It is noninvasive and helps children to feel peaceful and safe.

At the end of the relaxation, ask them to smile to themselves without moving their lips and tell them to keep that smiley feeling inside, somewhere safe. Suggest that they stretch and turn on their sides and come quietly to a sitting position with their eyes closed. Alternatively you could wake them with a 'snuggle' from a cuddly toy, and, when you have done so, they again can come quietly to a sitting position.

From time to time it is lovely to share with the child what they enjoyed about their relaxation/visualisation time. They might also like to draw their experience, while older children may be able to write down what they saw or felt.

If the environment is appropriate, end your YogaBugs adventure by chanting 'Om' together three times, and then sit for a few moments together with eyes closed. Sometimes it is nice to sit back to back with your legs crossed and share the warmth and support this gives you both. See how this feels – you will find that difference in your sizes is not important!

Relaxation outside YogaBugs adventures

Having learned the valuable benefits of relaxation through their YogaBugs adventures, children will be keen to apply techniques to other situations in their daily lives. Car, train, bus, boat and plane journeys may be ideal times to encourage children to empty their busy minds and feel a connection with their bodies and observe how they feel.

It is good to ask the children to feel as if their bodies were made of rock and then of jelly, so that they release tension in the muscles. These opportunities then provide an ideal time to ask children to create in their minds a place where they have felt very happy and safe. Enquire afterwards what they enjoyed about it or what they would like to do there if they could magic themselves into that situation now.

Children may also like to share what they have learned with their parents or other family members. It's interesting to try out when parents return tired and rather 'stressy' after work or at the end of the day.

Alternatively, these simple techniques are useful to help children feel focused before school tests or during panic or asthma attacks, or to overcome fears such as that of spiders and wasps. Combined with easy deep-breathing techniques, they can work well to help children feel stronger and more able to deal with challenging situations.

Chapter 3
YogaBugs Adventures

You have read why your child should do yoga; you are now familiar with the benefits. So this section is where the fun starts! It is most rewarding to do the story together and the pictures act as helpful reminders of what you need to do!

My suggestion is that you have a brief read through the story first so that you have an overview of the structure, which will develop your enthusiasm and storytelling ability!

There is a brief summary of the adventure at the start of each story. This also highlights some of the benefits that the child will gain from taking part.

WHAT IS YOGABUGS ALL ABOUT?

This is a helpful little introduction to share with your child and helps them to understand that, even though the adventures are wild and fun, they will, through yoga, learn how to look after their bodies, find peacefulness when they need it and develop strength and flexibility in their muscles.

YogaBugs come from a unique place; there is actually one deep inside all of us but not everyone can find it. YogaBugs like meeting each other and going on exciting adventures together. This section of our book is devoted to some of our stories and the wild and wonderful things that they enjoy.

Read the following together with your child.

YogaBugs is about:

* not trying to be like other people, but being me;

* being kind to my body and feeling happy, as I do when my friend makes me laugh;

* making me feel peaceful and floppy like that special time before I go to sleep;

* making my body strong and opening up spaces so that I can run fast, jump high and do roly-polys;

* helping me to stay bendy and do things big people can't do;

* making my body work well when I do my sport because it makes my legs, arms and body strong;

* breathing well, eating lots of fruit and veggies and enjoying every day;

* knowing when I feel tired and my body needs to have a rest;

* helping me to enjoy special thoughts and feelings instead of rushing to do the next thing;

* balance, which makes me move more carefully and not fall over;

* helping my body to feel good inside and outside and to learn about how it works; and

* helping me to see the sun, the moon and stars, to feel the grass under my feet, to smell the flowers and to play and have adventures.

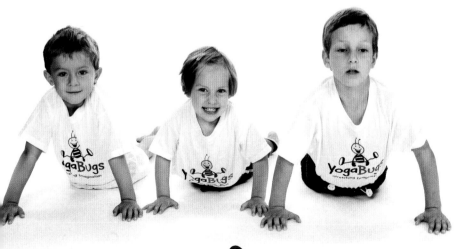

SummerHoliday Dream

This story starts as a conventional way of preparing for our holidays, packing all our favourite things and putting on our sun cream. However, things change somewhat when our taxi arrives as a flying car! We get caught in a cloud and make our get away as Superheroes. Luckily, we land close to a cave where we nearly jump out of our skin when we come face to face with a lion. He's delighted to see us and together we fly down to the African plains to meet all his old friends and family. Hector had been stuck in a cave in the dark for some time. We were able to help him out with our special candle and magic friends.

The postures

Candle

Bumpy Truck

Bow

Lion

Tent

Tree

Magic Bird

Cobra

Camel

Mouse

Aeroplane

The story

It's a beautiful shiny day, the sun is out, the sky is so blue and we are off on our summer holidays. But this is a dream, so all sorts of crazy things could happen to us!

Before we go, we need to pack our suitcases.

Let's sit with our legs outstretched and reach up with both hands to get the suitcase from the highest shelf.

Now we need to make sure that we take important things with us.

Binoculars, which are in the drawer behind us (sitting twist with legs outstretched), and sun cream (sitting twist the other way). Let's put it all over our bodies (gentle tapping motion over the whole body, head, chest, arms and legs and soft action on the face).

We need to remember to massage it into our ears, and rub the cream really well into our cheeks, too. (Make an O shape with our mouths).

Now let's give our favourite toy a big hug and put it in the suitcase as well. We don't want our clothes to get all scrumpled up, so we should make sure that we spread out our clothes (swimming trunks, towels and sun hat) flat in the case. (Crossed-legged and stretch forward.) Let's pop a **Candle** in for when we sit out on the warm summer evenings.

Candle

Now we can reach up and shut our cases and get ready to go to the beach. We ought to have a snack. So we have toast and jam before we go. Squat down and put the bread in the toaster. When it pops up do a star jump or two. Let's spread lots of butter (legs out straight in a sitting position) and chop up the cheese (using a chopping action with our arms). Now we can lean forward and munch it all before we go.

Boris, our taxi, has arrived with his **Bumpy Truck**, but this time it's rather a different one – this car flies! That is so cool. I bet our friends don't go in flying cars like this.

Let's fly with Boris and lean over this way and then lean over that way (like a magic carpet) and lean forward as we head towards a cloud.

Bumpy Truck

The problem is that we can't get out!
We are well and truly stuck in this cloud!
We are meant to be going on our summer
holidays and here we are in the middle
of a cloud and going nowhere! We hear a
deep voice from the middle of the cloud.
'YogaBugs, you have entered my cloud
without my permission. Now you will have
to come with me.'

'Oh, what are we going to do?' The cloud
is taking us to the top of a mountain
and it is going to drop us down on to it.
Get ready everyone, we're going to be
Superheroes: lying on our front and with
our arms out to the side and our legs
lifting up behind us, we can fly! This is so
cool. And look! We can
turn in the air (**bow**
pose and rolling on to
each side).

Now that we have
landed (rock and
roll) we should check
out where we are.

Bow

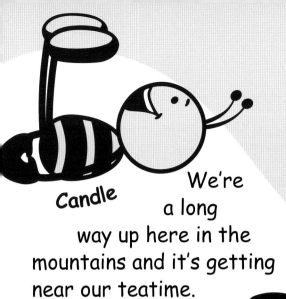

Candle

We're a long way up here in the mountains and it's getting near our teatime. 'Look, there's a cave (**Tent**) in the side of the mountain,

Tent

let's walk through the sticky mud at the entrance and go inside. Luckily, we've have brought a **Candle**, which will help us to see in the dark. We'll light our candle (rowing action with the leg on both sides) by striking the match.

Suddenly out of the darkness comes a loud roar – it's a **Lion**. We star-jump in fright.

Lion

'I'm so sorry I scared you, but I've been stuck in this cave for a long time and all I want to do is find my friends down in the plains below. I've run out of interesting songs and there's not much to eat. I can't see in the dark, and, now you've arrived with all your lovely candles, perhaps we can leave together. By the way, my name is Hector. Are you the famous YogaBugs?'

'Well, we don't normally speak to lions, and actually we're rather scared of you, but, if we can help with our **Candles**, then we would be so happy to take you down to where all the **Trees**, animals and birds are. In

Trees

Magic Bird

fact, we have a **Magic Bird** friend who might even fly us down there.' (Whistle to call him.) Mystic the Magic Bird appears.

All the animals are so pleased to see Hector the Lion back with them. Slith the snake (**Cobra**)

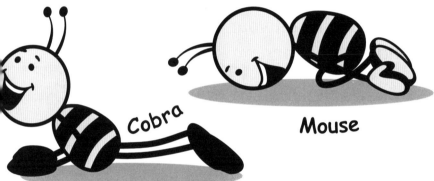

Cobra

Mouse

slides along and hisses a big smile. The three Grumpy **Camels** even manage to smile, too, and so does Mavis the little **Mouse**.

Now we need to think how we are going to get home. I wonder if Boris has managed

Camels

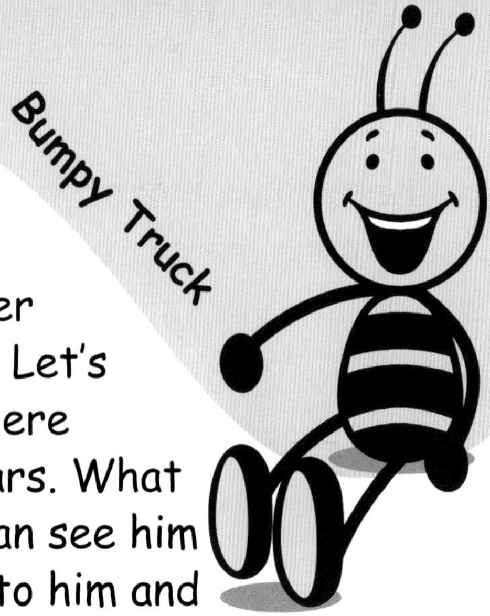

to drive his **Bumpy Truck** out of that rather unfriendly cloud! Let's have a look up there with our binoculars. What a bit of luck! I can see him now – let's wave to him and show him where we are.

If everyone is on board we can strap ourselves in and set off home again in our flying **Bumpy Truck**!

What an exciting adventure! And we're really happy to be heading home. Let's wave at the **Aeroplane** as we go

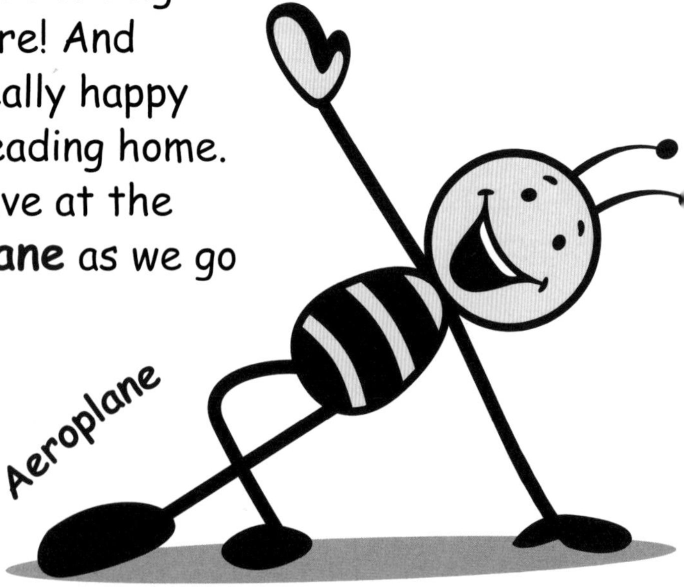

Bumpy Truck

Aeroplane

past and then make sure that we say hello to all the passengers on the other side too.

Relaxation

Let's lie down now and think about all the exciting places that we have been. Let's make our bodies feel heavy and relaxed and think about how cool it would be to fly up in the clouds in our car and then fly back down to Earth again on a magic bird. See if we can make this picture and feelings in our head and feel the soft warm wind on our faces and the sun on our backs as we travel on our beautiful dream adventure.

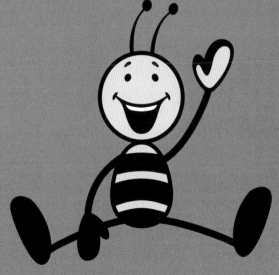

HUBERT
the Shockingly
Shy Giant

YogaBugs meet Hubert, the Shockingly Shy Giant. He doesn't have many friends because he lives in a scary big house at the top of a gigantic hill. He is angular, awkward and so very tall that no one can ever speak loud enough for him to hear them. Talking to him is a risky business anyway because he has such big feet and rather bad eyesight and tends to tread on visitors to his house before he actually meets them.

We need to make sure that we get to meet him, don't get trodden on and manage to make him feel very happy in himself so that he makes more friends to play with.

Highlighted in this story is the importance of kindness and helpfulness to each other and, through these gestures, we can help other people feel better too.

The postures

Snake
Cat
Bicycle
House
Deer
Horse
Windmill

Half-Handstand
Chair
Crab
Bow
Dinosaur
Mouse

The story

This warm-up is fun with your child's favourite nursery rhyme or a dance track.

Let's start by standing up and shaking all of our body so that we feel warmed up and ready for what lies ahead. Let's shake our feet and rotate them around. Now shake our legs – and really shake them. Now we come to our hands and make circles with them, then shake them and our arms too. Let's shake our head and now our whole body.

We may need to crawl through a hole in the skirting board so shall we do Slith the **Snake** (or Mildred the **Cat)** together a few times and then repeat it with all their noises.

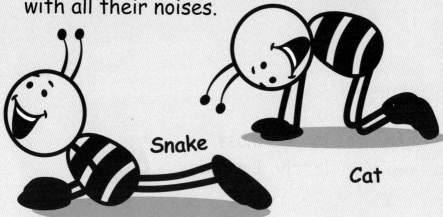

Snake

Cat

A great big bowl of energising porridge might help us on our way. (Sit crossed-legged and make big stirring motions and then change cross on legs and repeat the other way.)

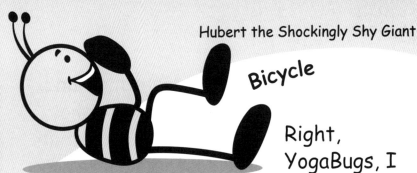

Bicycle

Right, YogaBugs, I reckon we are ready to meet this shy old giant. Let's get on our **Bicycles** and head off up the hill. We need to go slowly to start and then hold as we take a corner and then we begin to climb up the hill and then hold around another corner at the top.

Phew! Look at the size of Hubert's **House**! It is such a big place for one person – he must get very lonely. I wonder what our best way is to meet Hubert, because we want him to hear us and we certainly don't want to get trodden on!

House

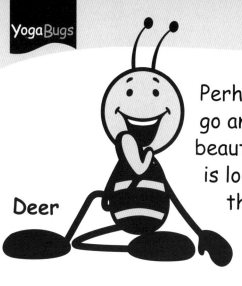

Deer

Perhaps we should go and talk to that beautiful **Deer** that is looking out over the hills and valleys. As we approach, she turns to look at us. 'Hello, we are YogaBugs and we have come to meet Hubert, but we don't want to get squashed!'

'I'm Deirdre! Well, you could call Romeo, the **Horse** – he's big, strong and powerful, and Hubert is very fond of him,' she replied. Let's call him: 'Romeo! Romeo!'

Horse

There he is, guys, up in front of the **Windmill**. Romeo loves to let people ride on his back and tells us to hop up and hold on tight.

When we get to Hubert's front door, there is no reply. We need to push (from

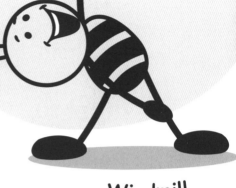

Windmill

Half-Handstand), but of course we are not strong enough. We thank Romeo for his help and decide that we should crawl in through a little hole in the wall and

Half-Handstand

pop out like Slith the **Snake** on the other side.

Snake

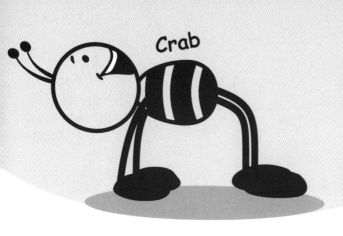

Crab

Chair

We have appeared in Hubert's kitchen. There is an enormous **Chair**, and a huge table (**Crab**). And look at that bowl (**Bow**) of crunchy giant nuts!

At that moment we hear huge steps coming down the corridor (**Dinosaur**). Let's dive into the crunchy giant nuts (standing forward bend) and hide at the bottom (Mavis the **Mouse**).

Bow

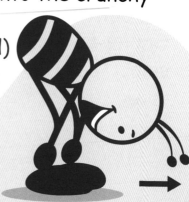

Dinosaur

38

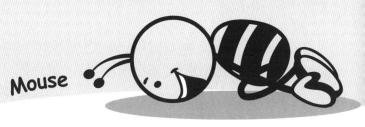

Mouse

Hubert sits down and we star-jump out of the crunchy giant nuts! Hubert is astonished to see us!

'We've come to help you and to teach you some of the things we can do so that you can see better, hear well again and bend down and talk to smaller people like us who come to visit you.' Hubert looks suitably stunned!

We show Hubert our clever eye exercises. We look up, down, this way and that way, and then we rub our hands together and put them over our eyes. Now we massage our ears from the very top to the very bottom, and that makes us feel calm all over. Sometimes we tell our grown-up friends to do this when they look a bit frazzled!

The best bit is to make Hubert all bendy like us, so let's take him through our Sun Salutation and see if he can reach the sky. (Hello, Sun, hello, Earth. (Tell Hubert he can bend his knees so that his hands touch the floor.) Beep-beep, woof-woof, hissy scary snake, woof-woof, beep-beep, hello, Earth, and hello, Sun. Now let's do the other leg.) Now Hubert doesn't feel shy at all.

Hubert loves it. He feels so much better and so much happier because, now he can bend down to talk to new friends, he can see them and enjoy playing their games with them. He gives us a giant smile and we all laugh together.

We say goodbye to Hubert and hop back on our bikes and whiz swiftly down the mountain.

Relaxation

Let's lie on our backs in the warm sunshine now and feel very pleased at how happy our Shockingly Shy Hubert has become. We feel the warm earth and grass under our bodies and the soft breeze and late-afternoon sunshine on our faces. Let's imagine looking up at the blue sky and see the funny shapes that the clouds make above us.

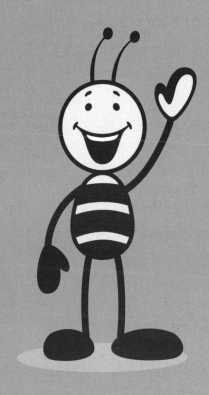

Where Does Everyone Go When it Snows in the World?

This story
helps us to learn more about living in the snow and how different animals and people manage it in their lives. Some of us have seen snow before and others have never seen it. Our adventure will take us to visit all the little and large creatures around the world who live in and love the snow and ice.

The postures

Dog	Snake
Cat	Frog
Bear	Turtle
Boat	Butterfly
Fish	Mouse
Lion	Penguin
Magic Bird	Skiing

The story

We are going to do a special warm-up exercise to get us in the snowy mood and we start with our feet together and standing up tall. Remember to keep our shoulders and our ears as far apart as we can because they are not very happy getting too close.

Let's breathe in and arch back and say, 'Hello, snow,' and then bend forward and say, 'Hello, ice.' Now we breathe in and take one foot back and bring our hands together above our heads as we rest on one knee.

This shape is like a pointed icicle hanging off a rock. Now we breathe out and take the other foot back and do a huge deep woof like a St Bernard snow **Dog**. Breathe in and let us lower our bodies to all fours like a

43

Dog

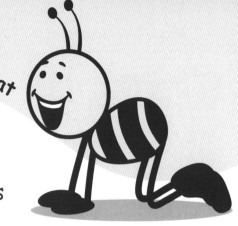

Cat

snow leopard (**Cat**). Now we breathe out and push our shoulders to the sky so that we look scary. Now curl our toes underneath us and push back to that huge St Bernard snow **Dog** and woof. Step one foot forward and stay on your back knee and be an icicle again; and then step the other foot (forward bend) and say hello ice, breathe in and reach up and say, 'Hello, Snow.' Let's do it again.

If we were to start our journey at the top of the world in the north pole, the creature that we might easily meet could be a polar **Bear**. These are actually huge, and, even though they are white and fluffy, they can be

Bear

quite scary if you meet them. Their babies are tiny when they are first born. They look like little mice and then like little balls of white fluff when they come out from the snow. They spend the early part of their lives all snuggled up next to their mummy in a snow hole. When they slide down the snow for the first time they often look like this (**Boat** pose)!

Boat

Lots of animals, insects and other creatures sleep when it gets too cold because this way they save their energy and they don't have to eat. Often, it is too cold for them to find the right food, anyway, and, when there is snow on the ground, they can't reach it, either.

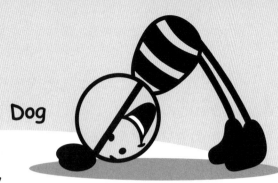

Dog

Now Mummy **Bear** is very hungry. She has been in the snow with her babies giving them warm milk throughout the day and night and she has not had anything to eat at all. She walks down to the sea and does the **Dog** pose as she looks down into the water and sees Matsy **Fish**. Yum! That'll do nicely! And she gobbles it up!

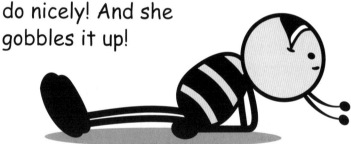

Fish

In Canada and Alaska, big grizzly **Bears** do this, too, and they like salmon. If anyone tries to get to their salmon before they do they stand up on their back legs and do **Lion** sounds.

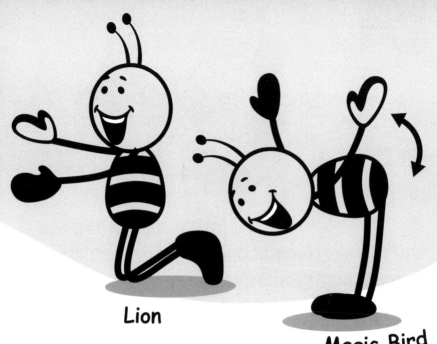

Lion

Magic Bird

When the days get colder, some animals such as birds (**Magic Bird**), head to warmer places while others get a bit more fur and develop special fat protection inside them around their very important areas, such as their heart and their brain. This special protection gives them energy and also helps them when they come out of their sleepy time and have to look for food.

Now we can also talk about other animals that hibernate or go to sleep for a long time in the winter. These can be found in

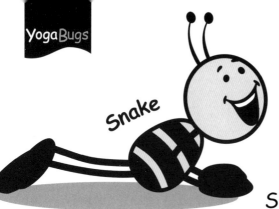

Snake

places such as America. **Snakes** like Slith crawl into old tree trunks with their friends and slither down into a warm comfy spot to sleep for the winter.

Nobby the **Frog** and his friends, like Slith the **Snake**, protect themselves from the cold by crawling into thick sticky mud, where they find they can stay warm and breathe through little air pockets in the mud. Talbot the **Turtle** and Teresa the Tortoise like to do this, too.

Frog

Turtle

When the snow begins to melt above them and the sun comes out, all the little creatures sleeping in the mud come up and say, 'Hello, Sun!'

In England, there are four types of Belle the **Butterfly** that go to sleep during the winter, and they are the small tortoiseshell, the comma, the brimstone and the peacock, so they must be very special.

Butterfly

They try to eat flowers and plants that have flowers on them as it starts to get cooler. Let's bend forward like a **Butterfly** munching on a flower.

Remember that **Butterflies** need to stretch out their wings before they go to sleep, as they will be still for quite a long time!

Mouse

Other very small things that like sleeping in cosy little places are dormice (**Mouse**) such as Mavis and hedgehogs such as Harold (rock and roll). Sometimes they sneak into our sheds, stables and barns to snuggle up in the warm hay. The other animals don't mind at all!

If we go to the bottom of the world now, we come to the south pole, where we might very easily bump into lots of very busy Percy **Penguins**. Even though there are lots and lots of them, they have a special sound that helps them to recognise one another.

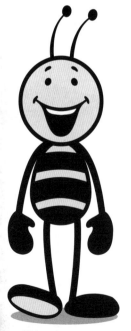

So, we've thought about lots of animals in the wintertime. Now let's think about some of the things that we do as people. We could go tobogganing (magic carpet), some of us might go

Penguins

snowboarding and **skiing**.

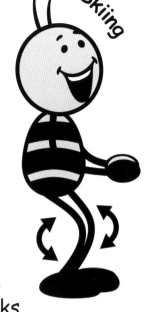

Skiing

Some people actually live in the snow all year round, and they are called the Inuit people. They build their houses out of snow and, even though their walls are freezing, they make it very comfortable inside with warm beds and lots of nice hot drinks.

Let's make ourselves a great big hot-chocolate drink. Sit with legs crossed and stir it well. After our drink we could climb into a big Inuit bed and cover ourselves with lots of warm blankets.

Relaxation

Let's try to imagine what it would be like to be a small animal surrounded by warm straw, hay or twigs. We can even make ourselves into mouse pose and see how nice it is to feel safe and quiet and imagine that we don't need to eat for a long time and we can just stay still and quiet and let our bodies keep us warm while we try to hear the quiet sound of our heartbeat and our breath.

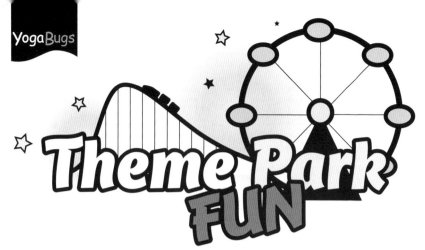

Theme Park FUN

This adventure shows the versatility of yoga postures and how adaptable they can be to so many different stories. This might encourage your own children to develop their own exciting explorations. We start off at home and prepare for our fun journey with snacks and stretches to get us in the Theme Park mood. We fly in hot-air balloons, twist in spinning teacups, rattle through ghost tunnels and ride the roller coasters.

The postures

Crooked Branch	Hot-Air Balloon
Baby Bird	Mouse
Sandwich	Rowing
Train	Camel

The Story

Let's lie on our back and squeeze our knees to our chest – we're going to be sitting for a while on the train, so let's make sure our backs feel comfy.

Let us circle our knees, holding each one separately, breathing in as we circle them out and out as we squeeze them back towards us. This stops our hips getting stiff too.

Now let's do **Crooked Branch** so we don't get tummy ache after eating lots of yummy Theme Park food!

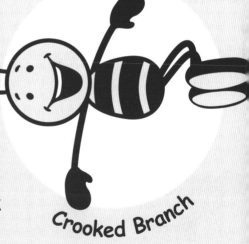

Crooked Branch

Rock backwards and forwards to prepare for some of the rides.

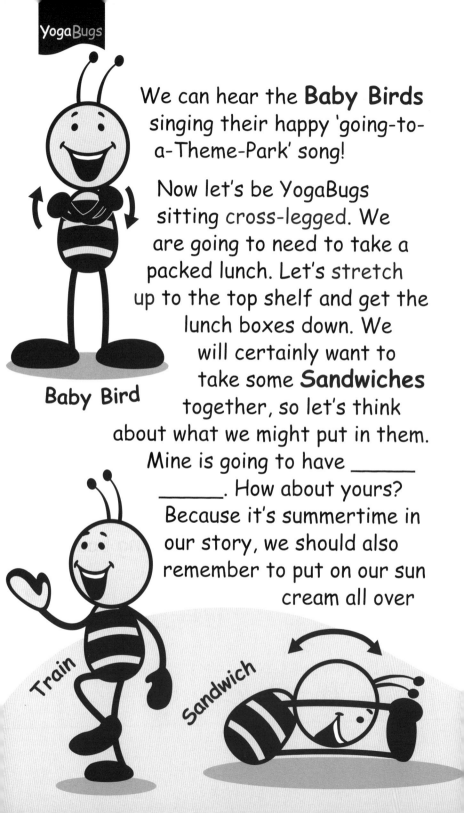

We can hear the **Baby Birds** singing their happy 'going-to-a-Theme-Park' song!

Now let's be YogaBugs sitting cross-legged. We are going to need to take a packed lunch. Let's stretch up to the top shelf and get the lunch boxes down. We will certainly want to take some **Sandwiches** together, so let's think about what we might put in them. Mine is going to have _____ _____. How about yours? Because it's summertime in our story, we should also remember to put on our sun cream all over

YogaBugs

Baby Bird

Train

Sandwich

our face, neck, arms, legs and body (patting all over body).

We're leaving on a **Train**, so follow me. Trains start slowly and gradually get faster and faster . . . Hold on tight!

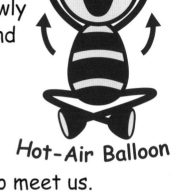

Hot-Air Balloon

Wow, it's hot here today (Hello, Sun). Gosh, look up there: it's a **Hot-Air Balloon**, which is coming to meet us.

Remember, we have to keep the helium gas going in to stay up (keep breathing in through nose and out through mouth).

When we come in to land (**Mouse**) we need to gather our things together and get into the **Rowing** boat, which will lead us in through the Theme Park gates.

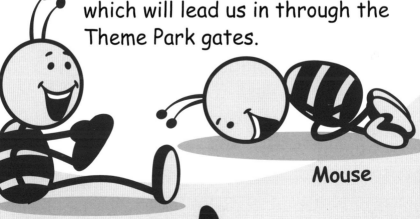

Mouse

Rowing

Look at all those funny people on stilts
(balancing on one leg and tiptoes)
standing watching us – they are clever,
the way they balance on one leg.

Let's skip now towards the spinning
teacups. (Sit cross-legged and rotate
slowly from left to right like washing
machine.) That's made us feel seriously
dizzy! Shall we sit still for a moment and
close our eyes and get our balance back?

How about a ride now on the roller
coaster (magic carpet). Wow! We're
leaning all the way over this way, now
back, now that way, now forward as we
whoooosh downwards and back up!

My shoulders feel very stiff after all
that excitement – let's give one another
a little massage.

I think we should all try
the log ride now! (On
our knees like **Camel**
and take arms

Camel

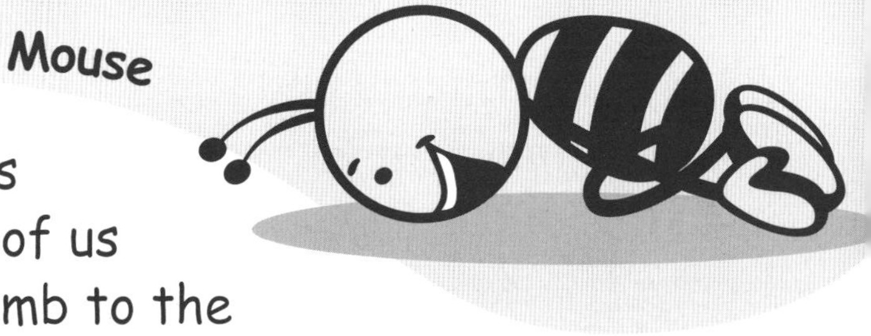

Mouse

forwards
in front of us
as we climb to the
top of the log drop. We
then come forward into **Mouse**, as we
splash down into the water. (Grown-
ups, take a handheld spray to spray the
children as they land – they will love it!)
Let's do this three times.

Shake and brush off all the water. **Let's
head to Space Mountain** (variations on
seated forward bend and boat pose).
**That was fun, but I think we really all
prefer the ghost train.** (Grown-ups, get
into downward dog and let your child
go through, and then you can try going
under them!) Don't forget to make
swishing, scary noises!

Sandwich

Let's have our **Sandwich**
now, because all this
excitement has made
us very hungry!

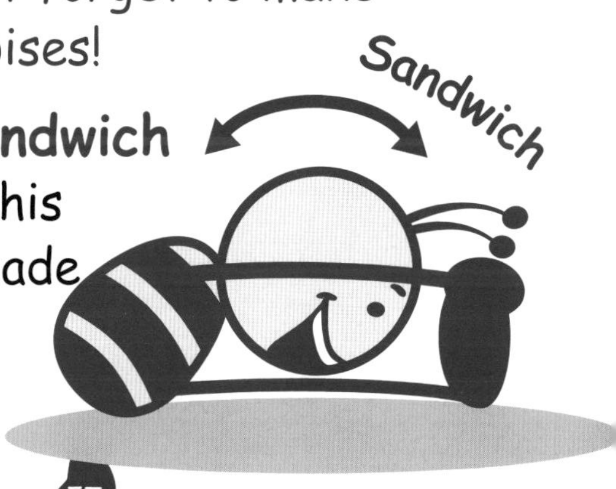

Gosh – what a day and what fun! How about a final special treat – a ride home in a helicopter (standing **Crooked Branch**). Here it is now, I can see it through my binoculars and it's dropping its ladder down for us to get in. Let's climb up and fly off (standing with arms outstretched and rotating upper body keeping knees bent).

When we get back, we hug everyone at home and do a drawing of our favourite ride at the Theme Park.

Crooked Branch/helicopter

Relaxation and visualisation

Let's imagine being snuggled up now in our beds. What a wonderful time we have had at our Theme Park. Let's spend a moment just thinking about all those exciting things that we have done. That log ride was something else and the ghost train was wicked! Just let's lie here for a moment or two and think to ourselves what our favourite ride might be and how exciting it would be. Now we're going to smile to ourselves without moving our lips and hold on to that happy feeling inside and take it away with us.

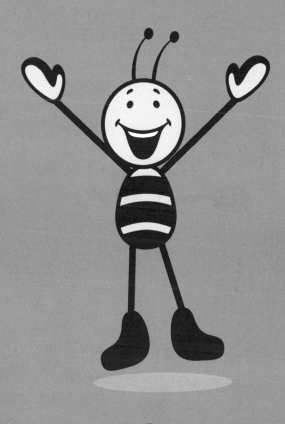

The Magic Pen

This adventure uses the powers of a child's imagination to create their own world. It has an educative element in it, telling them about different places as they journey with a baby swallow from South Africa to England where they reunite the bird with his parents. We make sure that we are fully ready to shape up for all the exciting things that we might see, be or do!

The postures

Sandwich
Penguin
Baby Bird
House
Magic Bird
Camel
Snake
Tree

Elephant
Lion
Flamingo
Rowing
Sphinx
Cycling
Boat
Dog

Surfing   Cow
Skiing   Rabbit
Bumpy Truck

The Story

Let's begin by sitting up really tall with
our legs crossed and then start with
warming up our neck and work down to
our toes. Let's stretch our neck this
way and now that way. Now we'll roll our
shoulders up to our ears and down. Let's
stretch our legs out in front of us now
and make a special delicious **Sandwich**
for our amazing adventure. Together
we'll think of really yummy things to
include that will help us to say healthy
and strong.

One day, a little
boy called Tomek
was looking out
of the window of
his classroom. He

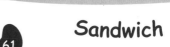

Sandwich

wasn't listening to his teacher at all: he was dreaming about what it would be like if he could magic himself around the world. At that moment he dropped his pen and bent down to pick it up (squat).

Tomek noticed a large piece of paper under his desk and decided to draw a lovely seaside scene.

Penguin

Suddenly, and to Tomek's complete astonishment, he was there at the beach in South Africa and there beside him were some Percy **Penguins**. Luckily he was able to understand them, as they twittered excitedly to him and walked in small circles.

They told him that there was a beautiful **Baby Bird** called a swallow, who

Baby Bird

had not managed to learn to fly in time. His parents had left to fly from South Africa to England for the summer and he was still stuck in his nest.

YogaBugs to the rescue!

Our little swallow is called Tweety and his nest is positioned on the side of a **House**, since this is a favourite nesting spot for these little birds. Tweety asks us if we can teach him how to fly. Let's show him our **Magic Bird** way of flying. Tweety is delighted because, now he is bigger and stronger, he can do it too!

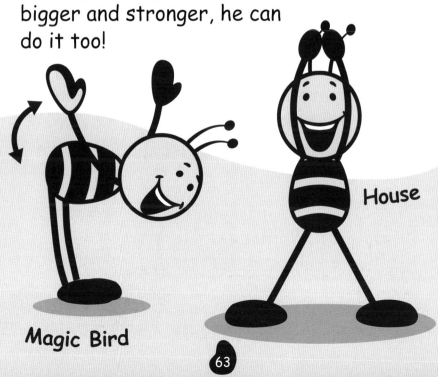

House

Magic Bird

Camel

We should try to find Tweety's parents miles away in England. But first we must fly over the deserts.

Gosh, it's dry and hot and there's very little water here. Some animals love the heat and have clever ways of storing their food and water on their backs in their humps. There they are now – a train of **Camels** led by Norbert! They seem to be heading to that large area of rocks.

Animals often find shelter from the hot sun by lying under the rocks, and we can see the tail of one there! It looks like a cobra **Snake**. We wonder if it's our friend Slith. We're rather glad that we are flying because this hissy cobra might like to eat little Tweety for his lunchtime snack.

Snake

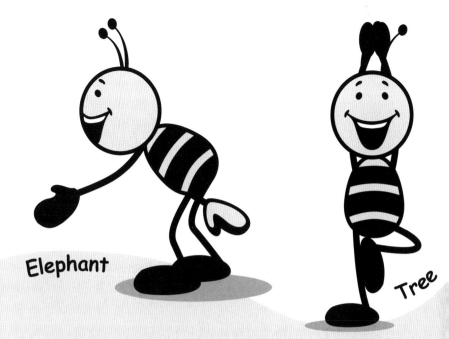

Elephant

Tree

Now we're flying over the African Plains with tall grasses and beautiful **Trees**. This is where we see the Big Game, the animals that people come from all over the world to see because they are so beautiful and in the wild. These include **Elephants**, who like to travel in long lines holding one another's tail. Let's try it too!

Lying there in the shade of the **Tree** are some **Lions**, the big strong Daddy lion, Hector, with his thick mane, and, next to him,

Lion

his small baby lion, Malice. They are too hot and tired to notice us today, so we will leave them to rest. All the animals that we have seen must have water to stay alive and often they have to travel many miles (or kilometres) to reach the waterholes.

Some creatures live near water all the time. As we look down now we can see a great clump of pink. These must be **Flamingos**, Felicity and friends. They are very elegant birds with extremely thin and long legs. Shall we try to do what they do? Remember if we wobble too much we might scare away the fish, which are our breakfast, lunch and dinner!

Flamingos

Rowing

We are leaving the Great Plains of Africa behind us now and looking down at one of the longest rivers in the world – it's called the River Nile. There is a family of Egyptians **Rowing** their boat in the direction of the famous Pyramids. These are places where very rich kings are buried and they are guarded outside by a **Sphinx** on either side.

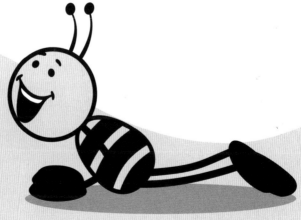

Sphinx

We are now nearing the Mediterranean Sea. Lots of people live around this sea and come here for their summer holidays. There are people swimming on their tummies – they can do a very difficult stroke called butterfly. There is even a family out on their pedalo (**Cycling**). It looks fun but rather tiring. There are some beautiful sails out there, too, on the small sailing **Boats**. We might just join everyone on the beach for a moment and relax in the sun (relaxation pose).

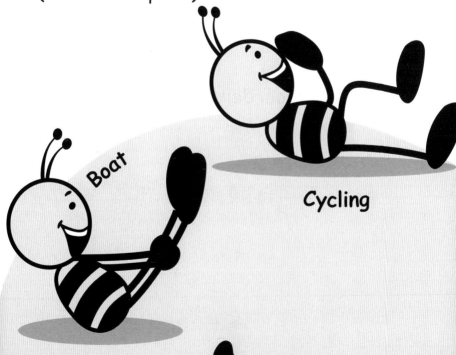

Boat

Cycling

We have come a very long way across the continent of Africa and now into Europe. There aren't big open

Dog

areas of space here, but there are lots of tall mountains and we are flying over them now. They are called the Alps (**Dog** pose) and they are in France, Austria and Switzerland. In the winter people ski and snowboard here, and sometimes in the very high mountains people can do this in the summer, too, because the snow never leaves these mountains. Let's join the cool snowboarders (**Surfer**). We can jump too and go backwards.

Surfer

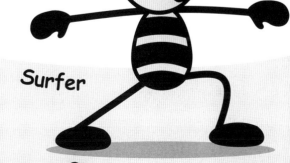

There are **Skiers** as well and they go very fast down the mountains. Tweety thinks that this is great fun.

Skiers

Now we are nearing some very tall buildings and one of them is the Eiffel Tower (**House**), which is an extremely large building in Paris, the capital of France. Some of us have been to France on our holidays. We say 'Bonjour' ('Good day' or 'Hello') to all the visitors who are standing at the top.

Tweety has loved his journey. He thinks flying with YogaBugs is very special. We are nearing the end now as we fly over the English Channel to England.

House

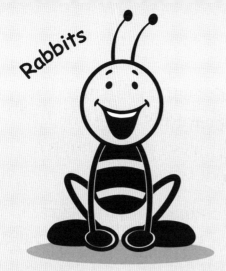

Rabbits

Bumpy Truck

There are the big **Bumpy Trucks** leaving the ferry ports and bringing all sorts of interesting food and drink to Britain. Down in the fields we can see **Cows** like our friend Mildred, and there are some little bunny **Rabbits**, Tabitha and Herbert, nibbling on the lush green grass.

Cows

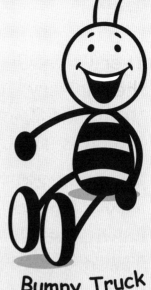

Baby Bird

It's nearly dark now and we see lots of other swallows gathering on the telephone wires and calling to each other (Baby Bird).

Tweety recognises some of his friends from South Africa. He calls back to them (**Baby Bird**). Tweety is so happy to be reunited with his friends.

Suddenly, someone clears their throat. Tomek looks up from under his desk. It is his teacher – he recognises her legs! Tomek looks down at his bit of paper under his desk and at the drawing of the seaside. He does a little smile to himself because he has been on a very special adventure and learned some very interesting things about the world that he lives in.

Relaxation

Let's lie down now together and imagine that we are on that beach with the warm sun on our bodies and the sound of the sea gently lapping against the shore. High above us in the sky is the shape of a small swallow. We know what a lovely time that little swallow is having, it might even be our friend Tweety. Let's pretend again that we are flying along with him and seeing the world as he does.

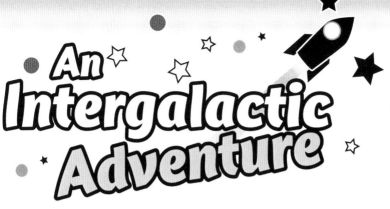

An Intergalactic Adventure

This story takes us into outer space, where we meet dinosaurs, cyber-men and surf down mountains on the moon. Our mission is to retrieve Jurij, our Russian Astronaut who has been left on the moon. He has missed his ride home in the moon buggy and he's frightened of heights! YogaBugs rescue him and together they ride back down to planet Earth.

The postures

House	Cobra	Surfer
Rowing	Dinosaur	Butterfly
Crab	Dog	Tent
Candle	Tree	Diamond

The story

Before we set off on our mission, we need to practise our Concertina Breath (four times) for special mission energy. We are going to be very cramped in our space shuttle and we don't want our shoulders to get stiff, so let's do some shoulder rolls. When we sit down for a long time, our hips can get sore, too, so let's stretch up and lean forward into a sitting cross-legged position.

Now, let's bring it all together with a special round of Sun and Earth Salutations (twice). Hello, sun. Hello Earth.

We need to make sure that we say goodbye to everyone at home (hugs). As we do so we see our spaceship (**House**) out of the corner of our eye and look at its giant wingspan (neck turns, arms out to the side).

House

We need to climb aboard (squat and sit with legs out straight). Remember, we must close the capsule and put on our earpiece (ear massage) and microphone (jaw massage).

It is very important that we check the control panel (seated forward bend) and joystick (**Rowing**). Oh, there goes the phone (ring, ring). We answer the phone, but we get cut off, and it rings again so we answer (other foot to ear). It's Headquarters. We have to go on an intergalactic mission as Time Traveller Secret Agents to save Jurij the astronaut, who missed the moon buggy back to Earth. He's scared of heights and wants to come home!

Let's get ready (**Crab**). Five, four,

Crab

Rowing

Candle

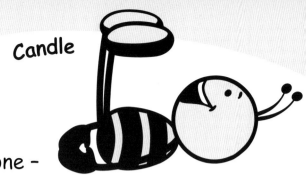

three, two, one – blast-off! (Sitting in wide-legged pose, stretch to right and left and extend forward.)

When we come in to land (roll back into **Candle**) we look out of the porthole (**Cobra**) as we check both sides of your spaceship and then peer out of capsule.

Let's lift up the capsule. Stand up (Hello, Space; Hello, Earth). Let's take a space walk from the capsule (looking from standing twist) with helmet on.

Quickly hide! We can hear terrible clumping sounds, like a moon rock.

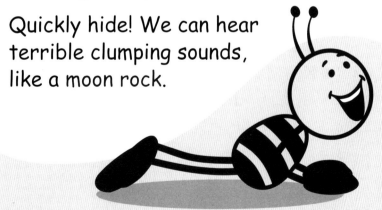

Cobra

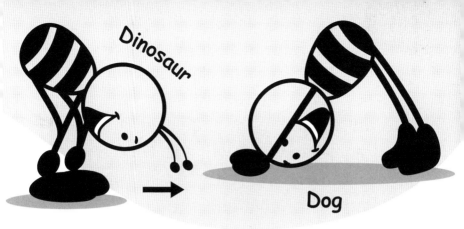

Dinosaur

Dog

It's a space-age **Dinosaur** and he's coming this way! Let's just pretend that we are moon Mountains (**Dog**) and maybe he'll miss us. Keep very still!

Luckily, he didn't see us. We are never going to find our astronaut unless we can see a little more of where we are. What's going on over there? It's the cyber-men. Let's do what they are doing! (Arch back and bend forward.)

'Excuse me, very important people. Could you tell us where we might find our friend Jurij? It's just that he really wants to go home now.'

They suggest that we climb that Moon **Tree** and now go a

Tree

little bit higher (other leg) for a better view. From there we will see where we need to snowboard (**Surfer**) down to a cave and that's where they last saw Jurij.

Surfer

Be careful, everyone: there's a supersonic **Butterfly** approaching. What enormous wings you have! And can you tell us if you've seen our friend Jurij? The beautiful butterfly tells us that Jurij is chopping wood in the back of the cave to make a basket for his **Hot-air balloon** back to Earth. Let's go and help

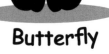

Butterfly

Hot-air balloon

him. (Make a cave tunnel (**Tent**) and let the children crawl through.)

Jurij is very pleased to see us but also very hungry and asks if we could make him some porridge. Let's get stirring (from cross-legged pose).

Now that he has polished off all the porridge, he would like us to start to blow up the balloon. Let's see if we can do it too.

The balloon is getting so big that it has lifted the roof off the cave and we can float out. Wow!

Tent

'Let's get in and see if we can float down to everyone back at home – they'll be pleased to see us and glad that Jurij is back.'

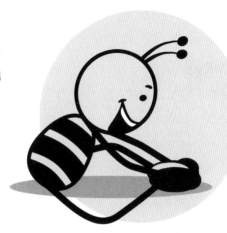

Come in to land (**Diamond**) Diamond and decide to stretch out in the warm sun. Jurij doesn't want to be too tired when he sees everyone, so we'll just have a little rest before we go home. Let's spend a little time thinking about our exciting adventure in space.

Relaxation and visualisation

Let's just think about where we have been and how happy we are now to be back on Earth. Let's allow our bodies to feel really comfortable on the soft warm grass and let the heat from the sun make us feel all happy inside. It's like that feeling we have when we know that something fun or good is going to happen. See if we can hold on to that feeling and take it away with us today. Just think about it for a moment and see how big you can make that feeling feel inside you now.

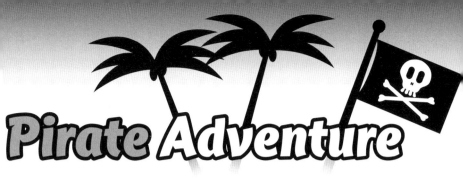

Pirate Adventure

We are explorers, adventurers and brave YogaBugs in this Pirate story. There's drama, excitement and heroes. Come and join us in this daring quest.

The postures

Mouse	Tent	House
Camel	Owl	Sandwich
Bridge	Plank	Frog
Crooked	Dolphin	Spider
Branch	Volcano	Snake
Boat	Dog	Mouse
Whale	Boat	Turtle
Shark	Tree	Lightning
Fish	Lion	Eagle

The story

Let's prepare ourselves for a high-seas adventure. We'll imagine that we are on a boat rocking and rolling (**Mouse to Camel**).

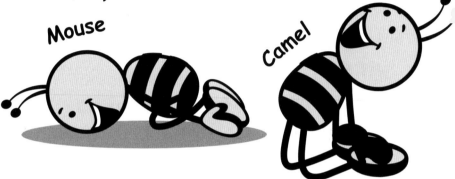

Mouse

Camel

YogaBugs have been given a special treasure map and we are going to go off to try to find the treasure tomorrow. But first let's climb into our big bed (**Bridge**) and rest.

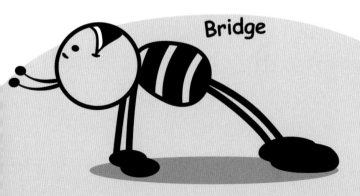

Bridge

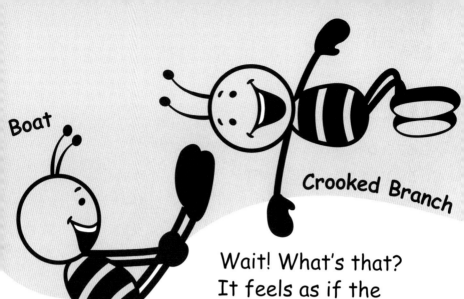

Boot

Crooked Branch

Wait! What's that?
It feels as if the
bed's rocking back
and forth (**Crooked
Branch**). Wow! Our bed's turned into
a sailing ship (**Boat**) and we seem
to be sailing on the high seas. Look,
over there, I see Whalley the **Whale**
swimming very close to some
big rocks. Right, then, crew, let's follow
our map. We need to get to Treasure
Island, so full steam ahead, Captain!

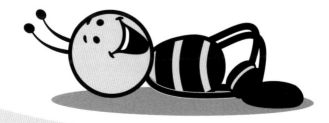

Whale

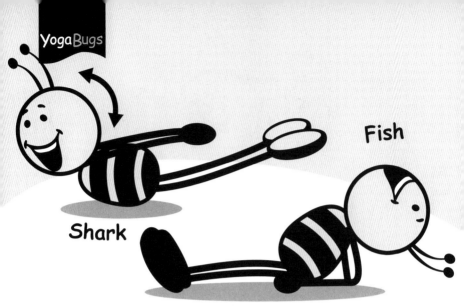

Fish

Shark

Let's peer through the spyglass – what can you see? I can see a group of **Sharks**, like our friend Brutus, circling around, and lots of strange-looking **Fish**. Oh, no! That looks like trouble. It's another ship with a skull-and-crossbones flag. That means Pirates!

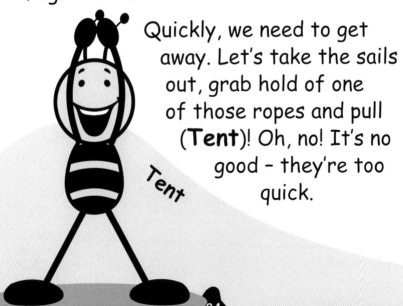

Quickly, we need to get away. Let's take the sails out, grab hold of one of those ropes and pull (**Tent**)! Oh, no! It's no good – they're too quick.

Tent

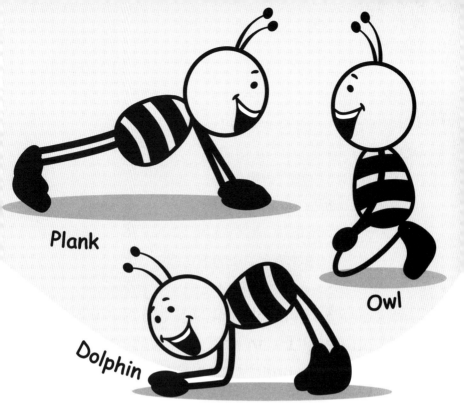

Plank

Owl

Dolphin

They are getting very close; I can even see one of the pirates with a parrot (**Owl**) on his shoulder. We might have to jump ship. Let's walk out on the **Plank** and jump into the water. Luckily, there are some **Dolphins**, like our friend Dolly, so they will help us but we need to swim to the surface (**Volcano**).

Jump on the back of the dolphins and off we go!

Volcano

Look, there's Treasure Island. I'm so glad we brought our waterproof map to find our way around! Be careful in this sand – it's really very deep and we have to do our sticky-mud walk. I hope it's not quicksand! Right, let's go and find that treasure.

Dog

The map says to walk over that very tall Mountain (**Dog**), and then row across the lake in the small **Boat**. Rowing now, everyone together. Somebody is not doing it right and we have gone around in a circle. Let's try the other oar (other leg).

Boat

We have to tiptoe through the forest of tall **Trees**. Watch out

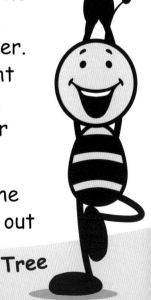

Tree

86

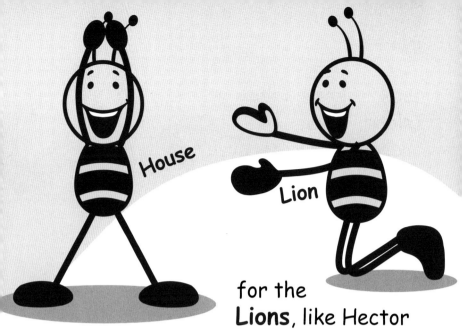

House

Lion

for the
Lions, like Hector
and Malice – we
don't want them to eat
us! And now, finally, we get to a little log
hut (**House**).

At last a moment to rest. Let's make
some **Sandwiches**. I am very hungry.
As we are a long way from home, let's
make a **Sandwich** with all the disgusting
things we dislike most!

Sandwich

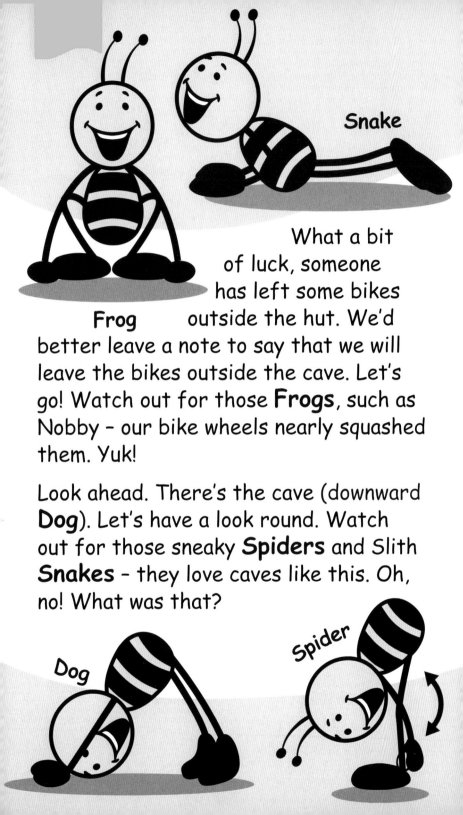

Snake

Frog

What a bit of luck, someone has left some bikes outside the hut. We'd better leave a note to say that we will leave the bikes outside the cave. Let's go! Watch out for those **Frogs**, such as Nobby – our bike wheels nearly squashed them. Yuk!

Look ahead. There's the cave (downward **Dog**). Let's have a look round. Watch out for those sneaky **Spiders** and Slith **Snakes** – they love caves like this. Oh, no! What was that?

Dog

Spider

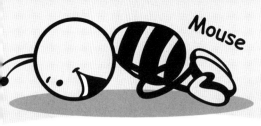

Mouse

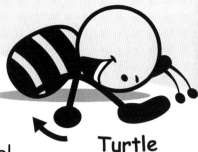

Silly YogaBugs, it was just Mavis the **Mouse**.

Turtle

There it is: the treasure! It is a big chest with a very heavy lid (**Turtle**). Look what's inside: gold coins. Wow! I think we should take the treasure and get out of here. I can hear a storm coming with Thunder and **Lightning**.

Hey, there are the **Dolphins** led by

Dolphin

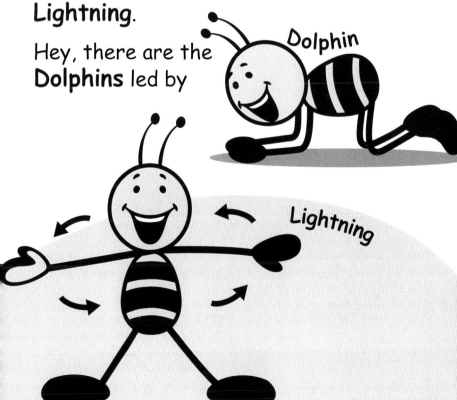

Lightning

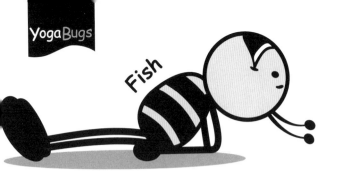

Fish

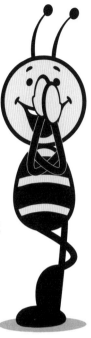

Eagle

Dolly and they're ready to take us back to our ship. Jump on quickly, because I can hear those pirates coming. As we hold on tight to the dolphins, we can look at all the beautiful **Fish** like Matsy below us and a magnificent **Eagle** called Engelbert, soaring above us. We really did outsmart those pirates and find the treasure. What cool YogaBugs we are!

Relaxation

As we lie down and rest now, let's think about our exciting adventure! One of our favourite memories was swimming with the dolphins, diving through the waves and feeling the warm sea and sun on our back. Let's see if we can feel now what that would be like by letting all the other things in our head disappear and by painting this special picture in our mind.

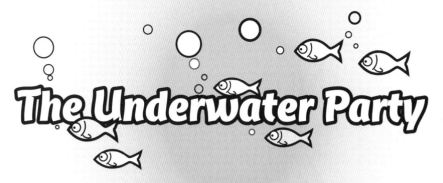

The Underwater Party

In this adventure, YogaBugs take on a very important role. They have been asked to find legs for a Mermaid so that she can dance at an underwater party. Mizzy the Mermaid is in a state of constant sadness because she is longing to join all her friends, but she wants to be able to dance as we do. We help her in her search and return successfully with the magic pearl that makes all her dreams come true.

The postures

Cat	Surfer	Dolphin
Dog	Penguin	Shark
Hero	Crab	Turtle
Baby Bird	Mermaid	Volcano
Magic Bird	Oysters	Rowing
Stork	Whale	Train
Tree	Fish	

The Story

We'll start from a sitting position and attach our head to a cloud with string to sit up straight. Now that we are feeling very tall in our backs and long in our necks, let's turn our head to the left, to the right, and then look down. We have got an action-packed adventure ahead of us, so let's make sure that our body feels ready by crossing our legs and doing a sitting twist, changing cross on legs and repeating.

We need strong backs for swimming and flying, so let's do **Cat** and **Dog** stretch and take away any tightness in our necks by doing **Hero**, with fingers interlaced and extended above head.

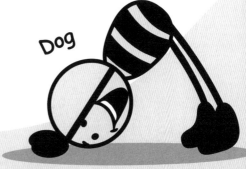

Dog

Hero

Today we are off to the beach! Oh, no, we're looking out of the window and it's raining (make action of rain falling on your head, face, body and thighs). Oh, bother! We're so clever, though, because we have a special spell to blow the rain away. (Cup hands and blow slowly out through the mouth.)

Cat

The rain has made the **Baby Birds** sing, because rain for them means that all the worms come up to get out of the wet earth. We look out of the window and see Mystic the **Magic Bird** on the windowsill. We open the big window and climb on to the bird's back

Baby Bird

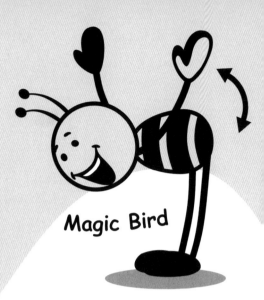

Magic Bird

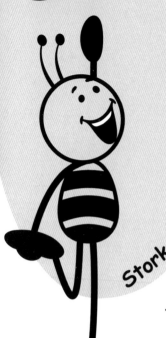

Stork

(**Stork**). Mystic the **Magic Bird** flies us to the beach.

On arrival we see the **Trees** swaying in the wind and then we walk through the deep sand towards the beach. Hey, wow, everyone! There's such a cool **Surfer**. He's so good he can even change direction! He's telling us to follow the **Penguins** to meet Cranky, the **Crab**. Cranky is very unhappy because he tells us that his

Tree

friend Mizzy the **Mermaid**

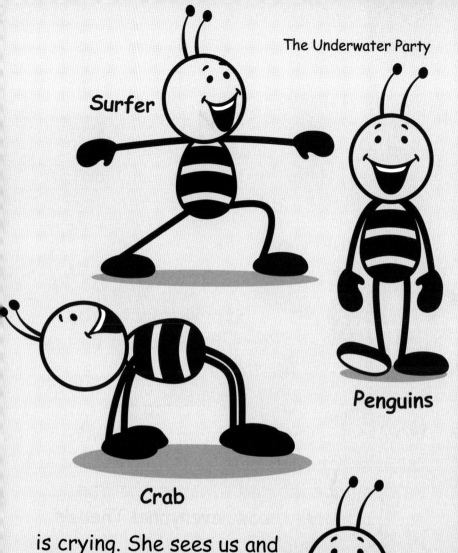

Surfer

Penguins

Crab

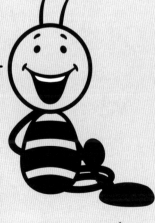

is crying. She sees us and turns the other way so that we don't see her crying. She tells us that she's crying because she can't dance at the Underwater Party if she doesn't have legs like ours. The only way

Mermaid

she can get legs is if she can be given a magic pearl that is hidden in an **Oyster** shell deep down under the sea. It is really too deep for her to swim. How do we get there, and who knows the way?

I know, everyone: let's ask Whalley the

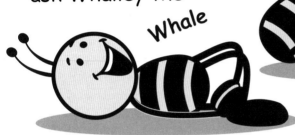

Whale

Oyster

Whale. He's so big and so clever. We'll ask him if he can help us, but, because he's so huge, he can't fit through the special tunnel that leads to the Oyster Beds.

Let's try our friend Matsy the **Fish**. Matsy is much smaller and can swim through very thin places.

Fish

The problems with the fish is that they can't remember which way to go because they forget everything so quickly.

I bet that Dolly the **Dolphin** will know. Unfortunately, Dolly is a bit of a show-off and all she wants to do is show us how she can dive through the waves.

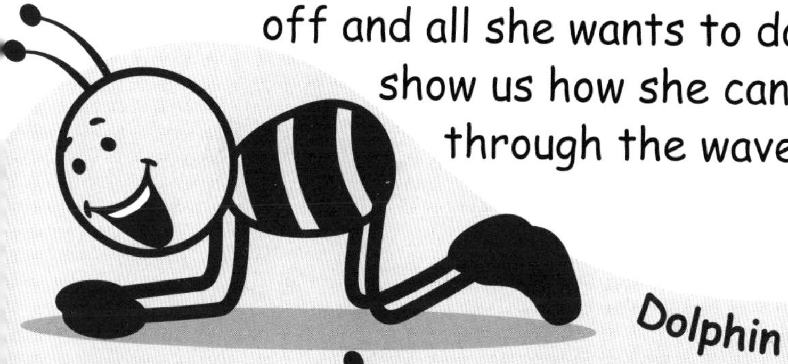

Dolphin

But she does tell us that, if we swim through the **Sharks**, we will get to the deep tunnel.

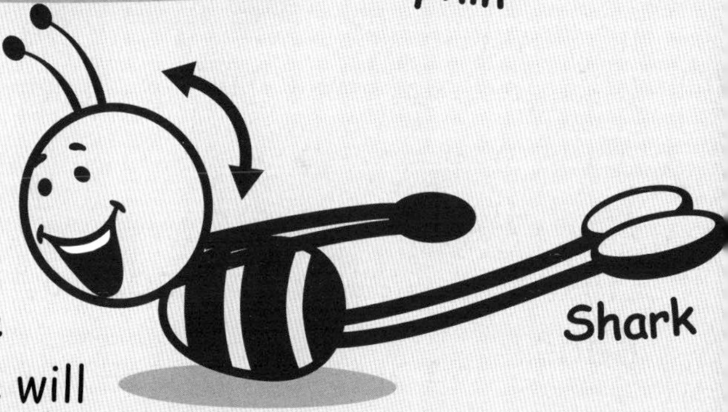

Shark

Oh, Golly! We're not at all happy about meeting **Sharks**, especially the notorious Brutus. They are so very scary and they might even eat us up for their lunch. Here's Brutus now! This **Shark** actually tells us he is really a friendly bloke and what he enjoys doing is just rolling along from side to side on the ocean floor. He does know, though, how we can find the tunnel to the **Oysters**. Wicked! First we have to find a rather grumpy Talbot the **Turtle**.

Dive down (forward bend). Grown ups can make a tunnel (**Dog**) and our YogaBugs can crawl through. Now we need to find that grumpy Talbot – don't forget to be really polite! He kindly points out where the **Oysters** are today. Now the **Oysters** are very private people indeed and they keep their front doors tightly closed.

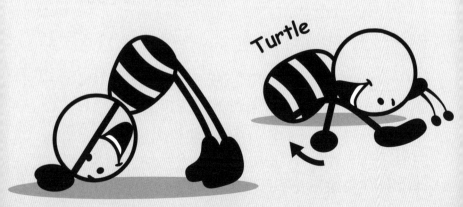

Turtle

Dog

Let's see if we can look inside their shells and find our special pearl for the **Mermaid**. This

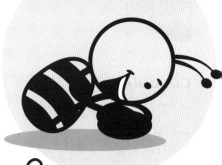

Oyster

special pearl will give her a spell so that she can have legs for the party! Yippee! (Pretend to look in lots of shells and then work with your child and pretend that the magic pearl is inside their shell!)

We take our pearl in our hand and swim to the surface of the water (**Volcano**). There's Mizzy the **Mermaid** now, and she's still crying. She turns away again so that we don't see her. She will be so

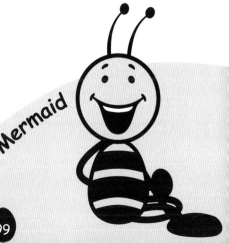

Mermaid

Volcano

pleased that we have been able to help her.

When we tell her the good news, she gives us two very big hugs and says how very happy we have made her. We tell her to have a really brilliant time at the Underwater Party and say goodbye!

Row

Now we had better **Row** back to the shore, because it's getting dark. Suddenly, the telephone rings and we have to answer it (foot to ear). We tell everyone at home that we are on our way. It rings again (other foot) and we tell them that we will talk about our exciting adventure when we get home. We get a ticket

Train

and get on the **Train**, which takes us all the way home. We creep up the stairs and hop quietly into bed.

Relaxation and visualisation

Let's imagine being able to swim down deep into a magical underwater world. Describe all the beautiful colours of the fish that swim past them, the funny octopus with all his arms waving at them and the incredible stillness of this underwater kingdom. Imagine mermaids swimming and sea horses floating by. Wake your child with a sea-creature puppet. Spend a few moments before the end of the class asking your child to describe what they saw or suggest that they draw or write about it.

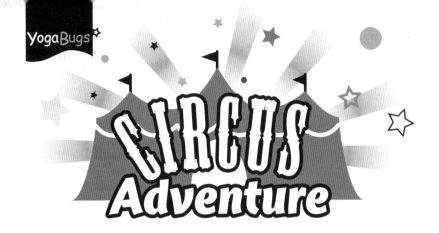

CIRCUS Adventure

The circus starts after our bedtime so we sneak out after dark, holding hands and taking candles with us. We manage to find our way into the circus tent and love all the excitement and fun. We do feel very sad seeing all the beautiful animals locked up in cages, so we decide to set them free and return them to their homelands and their families.

The postures

Sandwich	Tree
Candle	Lion
Snake	Deer
Mouse	Rabbit
House	Elephant
Tent	Horse
Monkey	Dancer

Archer   Plank
Magic bird   Bridge
Penguin   Boat
Candle   Rowing

The story

We're off on a night-time adventure, so we must make sure that our necks are nicely warmed up to make sure that we can see from all angles (lateral neck stretches).

Pack a suitcase (**Sandwich**) and remember to bring a **candle** to find our way in the dark, and don't forget a YogaBugs healthy snack and our night-vision goggles.

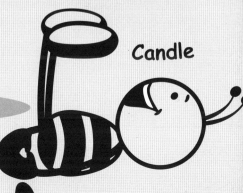

Candle

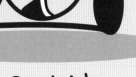

Sandwich

What's that noise? I can hear all sorts of funny noises. Can you? Listen carefully. What do you think it is? I think the circus has come to town! Shh, let's tiptoe over to the window, and look out (**Snake** pose). It is the circus – but look at their poster. The show doesn't start until after 9 p.m. That's past our bedtime. We'll have to hide in bed, and be as quiet as a **Mouse** so that everyone thinks we're asleep.

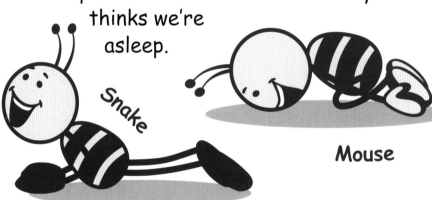

Snake

Mouse

Let's take nine deep breaths as we listen to the big clock chiming downstairs. It's time to tiptoe out of the **House**.

Close the door, and be as quiet as you can. We need to open the gate and of course remember to shut it behind us. Now we must all remember to hold hands crossing the road, and now we can run through all the thick mud left by the circus vehicles and hide behind the big circus **Tent**. Now no one will be able to see us.

It's so unfair that all the animals are kept in their cages. Perhaps we could use our special magic Bugs call to let them go free. 'We are the YogaBugs. We're special, that's for sure. If you would like to join us, we can unlock your door!'

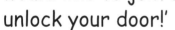

House / Tent

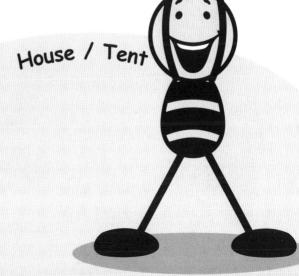

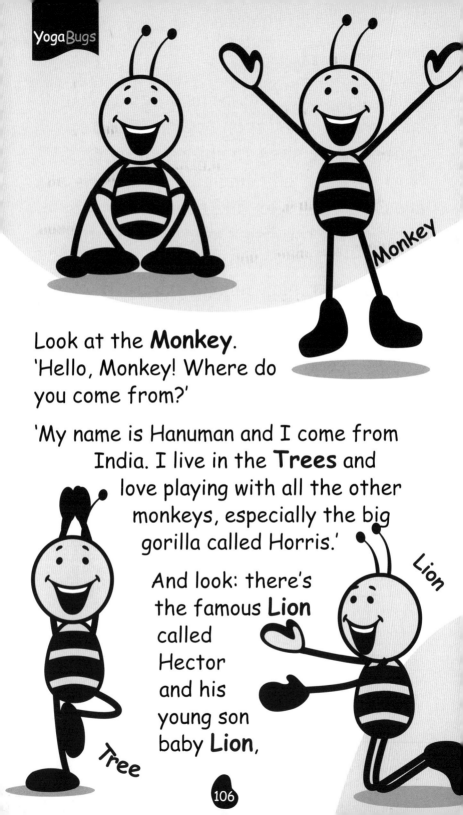

Monkey

Look at the **Monkey**.
'Hello, Monkey! Where do you come from?'

'My name is Hanuman and I come from India. I live in the **Trees** and love playing with all the other monkeys, especially the big gorilla called Horris.'

And look: there's the famous **Lion** called Hector and his young son baby **Lion**,

Lion

Tree

106

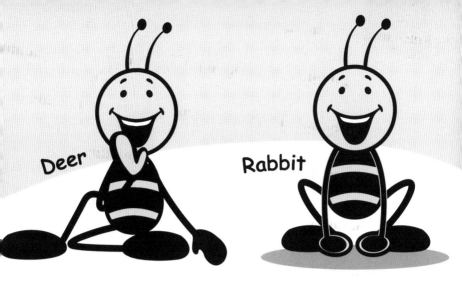

Deer

Rabbit

who's called Malice! Wow, listen to them roar!

'We came from Africa, where we ate **Deer** and **Rabbits** and rolled around in the sunshine!'

Gosh, I can see some very big ears over there! **Elephants**! Let's follow the biggest one, Ganesha, into the circus **Tent** and hold on to

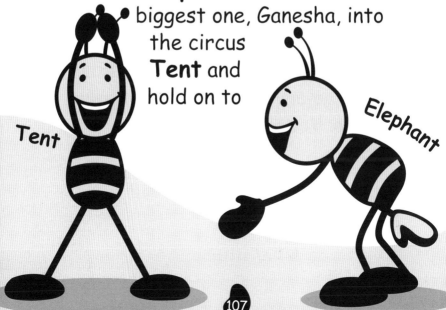

Tent

Elephant

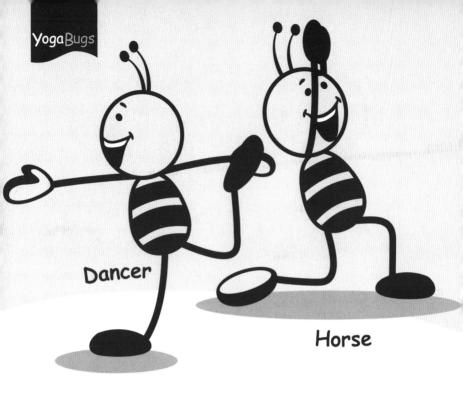

Dancer

Horse

the other elephants' tails so we don't get lost in the dark.

We'd better hide again or we'll be seen by the Circus Master with the very tall hat (arms extended to make a top-hat shape). Shall we hop on to the **Horse**'s back and go around the circus ring? What fun! Yee-hah!

Hey, YogaBugs, look what we can do. We can stretch our arms above our heads

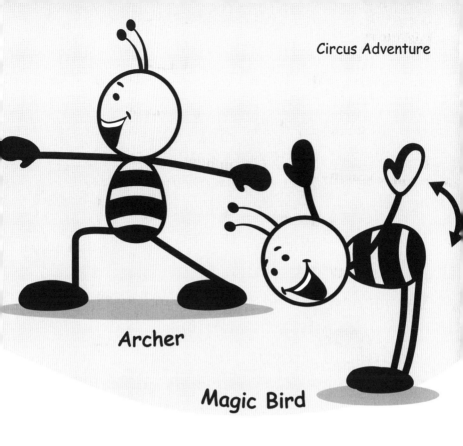

Archer

Magic Bird

and arch back. Now we look really cool and we can even copy those **Dancers** who are warming up.

There's an **Archer**, too. He can shoot arrows with fire on them – that's wicked! Let's copy him, and now let's try what those acrobats are doing – they love jumping and then squatting to warm up for their show! They can walk along the high wire too (**Magic Bird**)!

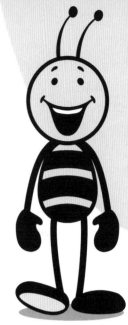

Who do we really like best at the circus? It must be the clowns. Look, they're coming into the ring now and walking like **Penguins**! Let's follow them round and see if they notice us.

My goodness! The lights have gone out. We must light our **Candle**. Maybe this is our chance to let all the animals go free. Let's unlock the cages, and put the **Plank** up so they can all walk down it. First we must repeat our magic spell. 'We are the YogaBugs. We're special, that's for sure. And

Penguin

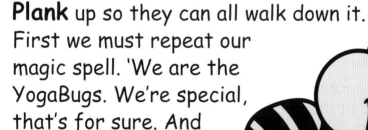

Plank

Candle

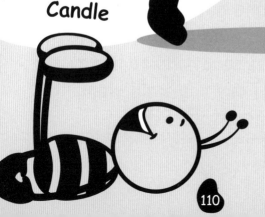

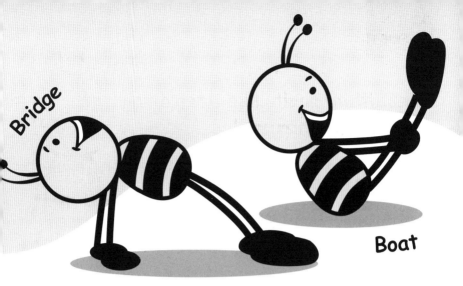

Bridge

Boat

if you listen to us, we can unlock your door!'

Quick, animals, run, run, go over the **Bridge**, and hide in the forest through the big tunnel of trees (downward dog). You'll never be found there. Wait by the river, and we'll bring a **Boat** to take you all back to Africa.

Rowing

There's the **Boat**. Have we got all the animals in? They are a heavy old lot in our **boat**, but let's start **Rowing** as quickly as we can. I think I can see Africa now with my night-vision goggles.

We'll make sure the animals get on to the shore safely and give them a big wave and hug goodbye! Now, if we close our eyes and imagine our nice snuggly beds, we can magic ourselves back there together.

Wow, what an adventure! I hope all the animals found their way back safely to their homes and their families.
I hope the circus master isn't too angry with us, but I think we did the right thing by helping all the animals to go back to where they came from in the wild.

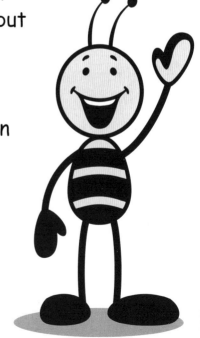

Relaxation and visualisation

Jelly or rock

This is a simple relaxation technique that allows the children to tense and relax their whole body. Start with the feet and legs. Instruct the child to lift one leg just off the floor and to tense every muscle they can find to make it as hard as a rock. Then let them drop the leg to the floor and make it feel like jelly. Repeat this process on the other leg, then tense their bottom muscles and their tummy muscles and arch their back and allow it to relax on the floor. Continue with the hands and arms, and hunch and release the shoulders. Finish by asking them to make the lion face two or three times to complete the relaxation process. Allow them to spend a few moments in total stillness with a very heavy body on the floor and their mind focused on the gentle sound and movement of their breath. Suggest that they think of how special it would be to be free if all they had known was being shut in a cage. How beautiful the world around them would seem and how big the sky would appear to be if they had never seen it before!

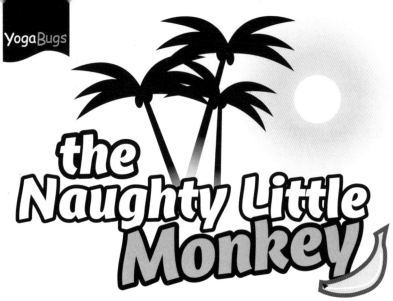

the Naughty Little Monkey

This story has quite a strong moral in it. There is a very naughty little monkey and his very naughty little YogaBug friend. Together they do some very wicked things. The other animals get really annoyed with them and decide to punish them for their behaviour. All is forgiven and friends are made again, but it is worth being nice to your friends or you might end up in a banana pit, too!

The postures

Monkey
Snake
Dog
Cat
Mouse
Butterfly
Tree

Crocodile
Elephant
Eagle
Lion
Cactus
Camel

The Story

Today, we're are going to learn together about a very Naughty Little **Monkey**.

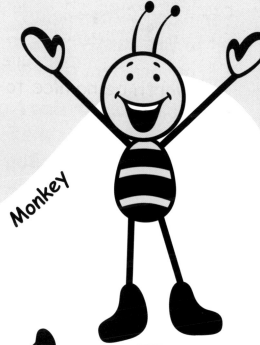

Monkey

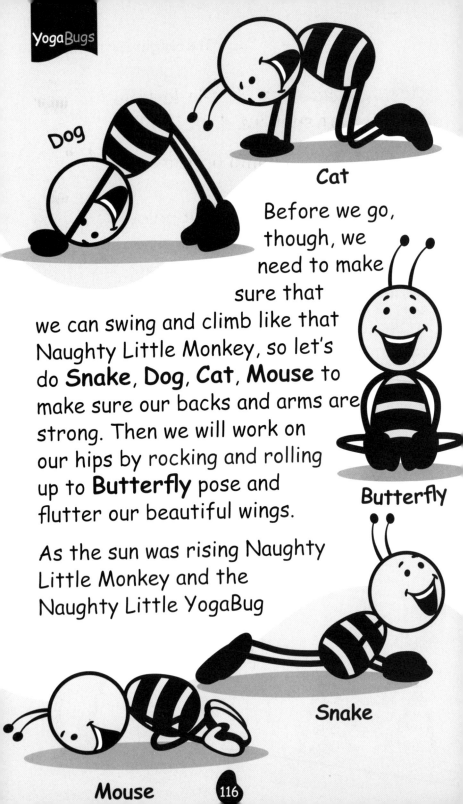

Dog

Cat

Before we go,
though, we
need to make
sure that
we can swing and climb like that
Naughty Little Monkey, so let's
do **Snake**, **Dog**, **Cat**, **Mouse** to
make sure our backs and arms are
strong. Then we will work on
our hips by rocking and rolling
up to **Butterfly** pose and
flutter our beautiful wings.

As the sun was rising Naughty
Little Monkey and the
Naughty Little YogaBug

Butterfly

Snake

Mouse

woke up and sang, 'Tra-la-la-la-la-la-la. What shall we do today?'

We decided to climb up the **Tree** and have a look at what was going on in the jungle below. We climbed a little higher to have a better view (**Tree** using other leg).

Then, we swung through the trees together and looked down. We saw Clik, a **Crocodile** lying by the river. We jumped down on to Clik's back, and made him very angry. He was so cross, he snapped his jaws and thrashed his tail.

Tree

The Naughty Little Monkey laughed and the Naughty Little YogaBug swung off through the trees.

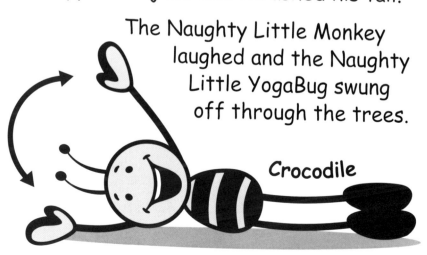

Crocodile

The next day the sun rose and the Naughty Little Monkey and the Naughty Little YogaBug woke up and sang, 'Tra-la-la-la-la-la-la. What shall we do today?'

Tree

We decided to climb up the **Tree** and have a look at what was going on in the jungle below. We climbed a little higher to have a better view (**Tree** using other leg).

Then, we swung through the **trees** and looked down. We saw a big herd of **Elephants** marching through the jungle. Ganesha and friends.

Wow! We thought what fun! We jumped down on to the Ganesha's back and decided to tie all the elephants trunks in a knot.

Elephant

Ganesha and the elephants were really angry (**Eagle**) and said, 'What did dou do dat for!'

The Naughty Little Monkey and the Naughty Little YogaBug swung off through the trees.

The next day the sun rose and the Naughty Little Monkey and Naughty Little YogaBug woke up and sang, 'Tra-la-la-la-la-la-la. What shall we do today?' We decided to climb up the **Tree** and have a look at what was going on in the jungle below. We climbed a little higher to have a better view (**Tree** using other leg).

Eagle

Then we swung through the **Trees** and looked down. We saw a big Daddy **Lion**, Hector, and Baby **Lion**, Malice, and we jumped down

Lion

on to their backs and pulled their manes. We wanted to make fun of them and they were very cross.

The Naughty Little Monkey and the Naughty Little YogaBug swung off through the trees.

The next day the sun rose and the Naughty Little Monkey and the Naughty Little YogaBug woke up and sang, 'Tra-la-la-la-la-la-la. What shall we do today?'

We decided to climb up the **Tree** and have a look at what was going on in the jungle below. We climbed a little higher to have a better view (**Tree** using other leg).

Then we swung through the trees and looked down. We

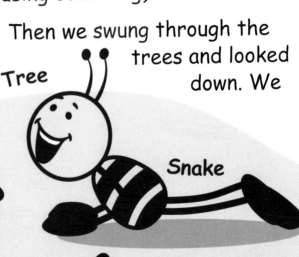

Tree

Snake

saw a Slith the **Snake** and we decided to pull his tail and make him cross. Slith the **Snake** hissed at us and told us to go away.

That night all the animals got together and decided that they would play a trick on the Naughty Little Monkey and the Naughty Little YogaBug. They decided to send them to the desert where the **Cacti** are sharp and the wind blows (**Camel** with arm actions to represent wind) while they dug a deep hole. They dug a deep hole in the jungle and filled it with bananas.

The next day the sun rose and the Naughty

Camel

Cactus

Little Monkey and the Naughty Little YogaBug woke up and sang, 'Tra-la-la-la-la-la-la. What shall we do today?'

We decided to climb up the palm **Tree** and have a look at what was going on in the jungle below. We climbed a little higher to have a better view (**Tree** using other leg).

Tree

We saw the bananas and decided that we might eat one or two. In the end we ate all the way to the bottom of the pit and we couldn't get out. We were very scared!

All the animals came and looked over the side (go through all the animals involved, and their names) and said they would help us to get out if we promised to be a good Monkey and a good YogaBug. We said that we were really very sorry for being so bad.

For two days they heard nothing and life

was a little bit dull. On the third day they heard, 'Tra-la-la-la-la-la-la. What shall we do today?'

Luckily, they all knew that he would be a good Monkey and that the YogaBugs would be good too and not do the naughty things that they had done before, but that they could still all have fun together.

Relaxation and visualisation

Jungle theme

I am sure that all of you know the story of Tarzan and those in The Jungle Book. Shall we imagine that we are like them and that we can talk to the animals and swing through the trees like monkeys. Imagine, too, that we can climb the trees as beautifully as leopards and swim in the deep African rivers as the crocodiles and hippos do. Imagine we live in a magical tree house high up in the jungle. We climb up special ladders to get around our house and we sleep on a bed of deliciously comfortable leaves. Think what a fun life we could have living deep in the jungle with animals, cooking our food over the camp-fire and looking up at the beautiful starlit sky. Stay in this special place for the next few moments and enjoy all the feelings it brings to you.

Chapter 4
Let's Talk about Balance

Balance in yoga is a very important subject and, now that we have tried some of the adventures, let's think about how valuable balance is in the postures that we do and also in our lives. Balance means harmony between what is going on in our heads and what is going on in our body.

Let's discuss what the word balance means to us.

YOGA POSTURE WORK

In our posture work, balance relates to pressing down into our feet in standing positions (like the roots of a tree). Grown-ups need balance too when they start to do headstands and handstands. You have to be a very good yogi to do these!

When we think about balance in our standing postures we also have to think about where we look. Generally, we have to look ahead – not up or down but just in front of us.

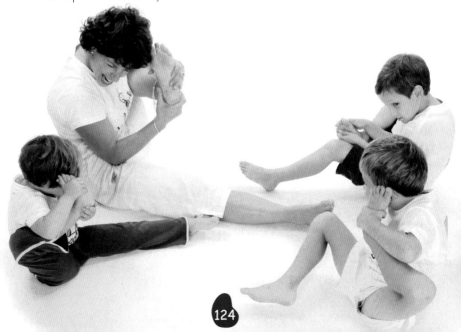

Let's work on some balancing postures that we have done where balance is through the feet:

Tree
Eagle – Engelbert
Magic Bird – Mystic
Stork – Lanky
Dancer – Darcy

Other balancing postures:

Crow – Beaky
Aeroplane
Boat
Camel – Norbert
Candle

Postures that mean that we balance our weight between the legs or on our hands:

Archer – Aimalot
Surfer
Tent

HOW DOES BALANCE COME INTO OUR LIVES?

We feel good when we eat a balanced diet. This means that we must eat lots of fresh fruit and vegetables as possible. Let's think together about what we know is good for our bodies. Food that we can help to prepare is much better than food that comes out of a packet or goes straight in the microwave oven.

We also feel good when:

* we take exercise and sleep well;
* we are not anxious about things in our lives, such as our homework or our reading;
* we don't have to worry about getting to school on time or being ready to leave for school;

*   we have all our stuff in the right place at the right time, such as our swimming kit and our PE gear.

Feeling free from worries helps us feel balanced, too. Also, when we spend our pocket money we like to feel balanced and happy with what we buy.

Balance is also important in our friendships. We feel sad if some of our friends just take ideas and things from us and don't share back in the same way. We like to feel that our friendships are balanced between giving and taking and about sharing.

And we like to feel that we have a balance between school life and time at home; time outside and time relaxing in front of the television or playing on the computer.

Relaxation

Balance comes into our lives in many different ways and it is important that we be aware of it and how we feel. When we don't feel good it is more than likely that a valuable part of our daily routine has been forgotten about. Let's take a moment to think about how we might be able to make our day-to-day lives feel better and more in harmony with the person we would like to feel and be.

Some fun YogaBugs games to share with friends

Box of Tricks
Get yourself a box of toy animals or put together a collection of cuddly toys that we use in the YogaBugs Adventures. It is fun to ask your child or children to put their hand in and pull out one of the animals. Their task is then to do the posture and make the animal face or noise. Older children might perhaps be able to tell you why it is good for them and what parts of the body it can help.

Musical Statues
Play music and when it stops ask children to get into a pose (tree, magic bird, stork etc.) and test them to see how long they can last without wobbling.

Put hoops or circles on the floor and ask the children to dance. When the music stops ask the children to find a hoop and take up a pose. Always have one fewer hoop than the number of children in the class, take one away until you have a winner.

In order for children not to get upset when they are 'out', ask them to join you on your panel of judges.

Jungle Game
This game is suitable for the older end of YogaBugs and is similar to Paper, Stone, Scissors, where children use the following animals: Snake frightened of Lion, Lion frightened of mouse, snake eats mouse. Crazy star jumps are the prize!

Divide children into groups of three and get them to play for a couple of minutes.

Chinese Whispers
This involves whispering the name of the pose and asking a child to demonstrate the posture at the end. Go in a circle starting with you and around to the last child. Then the last child does the posture. This could also be adapted to funny-face Chinese Whispers, but make sure the others don't see!

Grandmother's/Witch's Footsteps
Rather dotty grandmother deep in jungle turns around and all she can see is trees, crows, storks, houses, etc. (Each time the grandmother/adult turns around she/he says, 'All I can see is trees, houses . . .' or whatever, to which the children perform the postures and avoid wobbling and falling over.) This is always a very popular game and the children usually end up in fits of giggles!

YogaBugs Say . . .
. . . or Freeze and Unfreeze (like Simon Says). This is a fun way of testing out how much they know and is always a very popular game with all YogaBugs

Little Tricks

* Getting up without using hands.
* Jumping from knees to feet.
* Rolling from back up to feet.
* Marching and then going into a posture on instruction.

Clapping Game

This involves sitting in a circle, and each child is labelled as an animal and a clapping routine is established by the whole group. Each child has to say what they are and identify another animal while keeping the clapping going continuously.

They clap and say 'snake' and then look to Dog, and then the next child says 'dog' to Cat, and so it goes on.

Balloon Game

Children lie on the floor with their heads in a circle. They must balance a balloon on their feet and pass it around the circle. The object is not to let the balloon fall to the floor – and no hands are allowed! Excellent exercise for developing co-ordination.

Crab Football

Guaranteed to exhaust everyone! A great team game with friends and movement can be only sideways. Make sure you pass to the right team member! Grown-ups are the umpires!

Foot-Passing Game

Pass conkers, marbles or acorns to each other with feet. The object is to try not to let them drop. Excellent way of improving co-ordination. You could also do the foot massage in the list of postures. In addition, you could have an area with talc, which the children put their one foot into and then transfer it on to dark paper. The footprint will stay if you spray it with hair spray.

Mirroring Game

Use chopsticks or coffee stirrers to mirror each other's movements.

Musical Mats
Put a posture name face down, or for little ones draw the pose, and when the music stops they have to land on the pose and demonstrate the posture. You could then remove a pose until the last child wins or just make it a fun activity.

Animal Know-How
Allowing a child in the circle to choose a posture. Each child then has to add what that animal eats, where it sleeps and what sound it makes.

Passing the Chimes
This is a 'concentrating game' in which the children have to pick up the chimes or a little bell and carry them/it to one of the other children in the class. They must avoid the chimes touching or the bell ringing. This continues until you decide to end. The children really enjoy the challenge and their concentration is wonderful.

Candle Meditation (*Tratak*)
Ask the children to observe a candle and then hold its image with their eyes closed. This has a very quietening effect on everyone and is a basic introduction to simple meditation techniques. They look back at the candle if the picture fades when their eyes are closed.

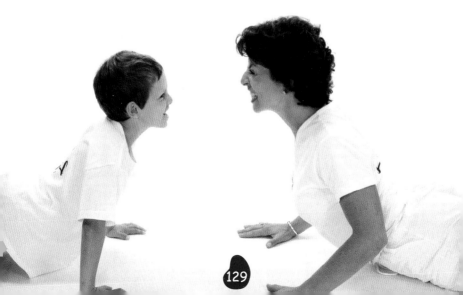

Chapter 5
Breathing Techniques

First, a short explanation: the parts that are written in bold below are for the grown-ups, while the instructions are written for the children to follow. Right, let's get down to some breathing.

Concertina Breath
An energising breathing exercise that warms them up, gets oxygen to their brain and helps them feel more active.

This is like playing a squeezebox. Interlacing the fingers under the chin, you then raise the elbows up and take the head back as you breathe in through the nose. You breathe out through the mouth and lower the elbows down and rest the chin back on the interlaced fingers.

Sithali Breath
This exercise is excellent in hot weather. It helps them to stay cool while enabling them to produce saliva and thereby quenching thirst (particularly good when you have temporarily run out of drinks on a car journey)!

You can either roll your tongue like a sausage or make an O shape with your mouth. The air is drawn in over the tongue and the breath out is through the nose.

Deep Breathing/Abdominal Breath
This exercise is helpful for toning the abdominal muscles, improving digestion and helping children to feel calm and focused. It is practised with the children lying on their back and breathing is in through the nose and out through the nose.

A useful way of demonstrating deep breathing is to place a small duck or boat on your child's tummy. As they breathe in, the boat or duck rises up on a wave and, as they breathe out, the object comes down. We don't want the toy to fall off, so they need to breathe deeply and evenly at all times, otherwise the boat or duck might find itself in a scary storm.

The Ha Breath
Both safe and fun, this encourages the use of abdominal muscles in preparation and also helps to energise and warm children up.

With the children sitting either cross-legged or on their knees, you breathe in together through the nose and let out the breath through the mouth to make a 'ha' sound. Often, this will develop into a lovely laughing session together, but it will also be fun to make the sound and observe the feelings afterwards.

Wind Blowing
This is a great contrast to the ha breath, because, while it uses the same idea, the out breath is slow and through O-shaped lips. This type of breathing stimulates the parasympathetic nervous system, which slows the heart rate.

Breathe in through the nose and blow out through the mouth. The aim is to get children to fill their chest with air and then release the air out of the mouth in a slow and steady way. Practise for only a short time to avoid dizziness.

Breathing techniques are very good for respiratory problems such as asthma and anxiety-related problems. We tend to use as little as a third of our lungs in day-to-day breathing. By learning to control their breathing and taking deeper breaths, children can improve their whole sense of wellbeing and their outlook.

Chapter 6
Warm-up Exercises

Again, the purely informative part for the adults is in bold, while the instructions for the children are given underneath.

Neck Stretches, Shoulder Rolls and Stretches
To release tightness in the shoulders and stiffness in the neck, and to warm up the thoracic spine.

Neck stretches: Sit cross-legged and make a space between the ears and the shoulders with a long straight back. Now take one arm (right) and stretch it over your head towards your ear on the (left) other side. Breathe in and as you breathe out lower your head to the right side and gently release any stiffness there. Repeat with the other arm on the other side. Try to count for six breaths.

Shoulder rolls: We take our shoulders all the way up to our ears and then we roll them all the way back down again. Sometimes, we feel some funny feelings inside but we know that we are helping to keep our shoulders working well. Do this six times and then encourage the children to move their shoulders the other way.

Eye Exercises and Palming
To relax around the eyes and increase space between the brows.

Sitting with your legs crossed and your back tall and strong, look up to the ceiling and down to the floor. Now look this way and then that way, and now back to the ceiling and down to the floor. Repeat the exercise a few times and then rub your hands together and place the warm palms over your eyes and count to eight slowly.

Ear and Jaw Massage
Acts as a form of body massage through the ears and takes away tension in the jaw.

Place your fingers and thumb around the top rim of your ear. Now gently massage all the way from the top of the ear to the bottom of the ear lobe. It feels really nice and relaxing.

Massaging under the collar bone can also be effective in focusing the children. One hand under collar bone, one on tummy. Improves thinking skills, promotes a sense of relaxation.

There are two little spaces under your collarbone and almost in line with your ears. You place your finger in one and your thumb in the other and gently massage. It can feel quite stiff under there but massaging is rather nice. With the other hand you can softly rub your tummy.

These massages should be done for about twenty breaths or 1 minute.

Rocking Horse
To warm up the spine and introduce motion.

Children and grown-ups enjoy this one. Lying on your back, hug your knees into your chest and start to rock backwards and forwards about ten times. It makes you feel ready for your next postures.

Butterfly
To open the hip area and strengthen the lower back.

From the rocking-horse exercise, your child can come up to a sitting position on their bottom with the soles of their feet touching and their knees bent. They love telling you the colour of their butterfly wings as they gently move their knees up and down. It is nice to conclude this exercise by bending forward to sip from a pretty flower. Children do this beautifully while it brings tears to most adult eyes as they endeavour to extend forward to the floor!

Rowing

To release the hip joints through breathing and motion.

Sitting with both legs outstretched, take hold of one foot with both hands. Breathe in as you take the foot down the opposite leg towards the foot and out as you bring the foot up the leg again and towards the tummy. Perform about ten times and then change legs. Children love answering the phone (foot to ear) or rocking the babies by cradling their foot in their opposite elbow and rocking. Remember to do both sides!

Cat and Dog Stretch

Bringing all the above together by releasing the upper back and shoulders, lower back and hamstrings. The combination also helps to focus awareness into the front and back of the thighs and knees.

Place hands under shoulders and knees under hips so that you are on all fours. Now breathe in and think that you are a really scaredy-cat by pushing your tummy towards your back and your shoulders towards the ceiling, and taking your chin towards your chest. As you breathe out, imagine pulling your head away from your tail and come back to your first position.

Now repeat, but at the end curl your toes underneath you, press down into your hands and lift your bottom up towards the sky. Push your chest back towards your legs and let your neck feel comfy with your eyes looking back between your ankles. See if you can make the same space between your hands and your ankles. Breathe in and, as you breathe out, come back to all fours.

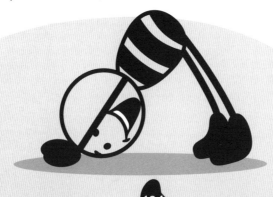

Cross-Crawling

Hand or elbow to opposite knee. This stimulates both brain hemispheres, good for reading, writing and spelling. It improves co-ordination, especially if your child was a bottom shuffler, not a crawler.

This is just what it says!

Sun Salutation with Cat/Dog Variation

Children enjoy the linking of postures with breath. Don't worry about whether they take their left or right leg back until they are aware of them. The accompaniment of sounds to each pose can also be great fun for the Bugs.

Standing in Mountain pose with feet together, breathe in and stretch up towards the sky (Hello, Sun). Breathe out and fold forward into Rag Doll (Hello, Earth) – for Rag Doll see Page 155. Place hands either side of the feet (bend knees to reach the floor if necessary), breathe in and step one foot back. This is Roadrunner (beep-beep). Breathe out and now take the other foot back into Dog (woof).

Breathe in and now bend your knees and your elbows and lower your tummy to the floor. Breathe in and start to make a hissy sort of face and a snaky sound (hiss) and then breathe out and push back to Dog (woof). Step one foot forward and breathe in (beep-beep) then the other, breathe out (Hello, Earth), breathe in and stretch up (Hello, Sun), breathe out and come back to mountain posture. Repeat with the other leg and do the sequence as many times as you feel your child would like to.

Chapter 7
Postures and Benefits

Once again, The postures and their benefits in this section are high-lighted in bold for the grown-ups, while the instructions are given in a child-friendly format.

Aeroplane (Vasistasana)
Strengthens wrists, shoulders, torso and thighs, can also be known as a rainbow.

The best way to approach this posture is from the Dog pose. We place the outside of our left foot on the floor and bring the right leg over, while raising the right arm towards the ceiling and turning (when balanced) to look up at it. Repeat on the other leg.

Archer (Virabradrasana II)
Tones abdominal muscles, brings flexibility to leg and back muscles.

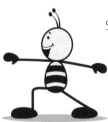

Step the feet wide apart so that wrists line up with ankles when we stretch our arms out. Turn your front foot out and our back foot in a little bit. Stretch your arms out to the side and bend our front leg while keeping the back one strong and straight. Let's see if we can make a line from our knee to our ankle on the front leg, then we will be a really cool archer.

Now turn and do the other leg, because YogaBugs can clap hands together to shoot arrows backwards and forwards.

Baby Bird
Helps to release stiffness in the shoulders.

We fold our arms and then place our hands on our shoulders so that our arms are crossed at the elbows. Baby birds talk to each other with their beaks and we like our elbows to work like a beak, which opens and closes. This can also act as a lovely hug.

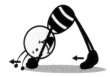

Bear

This is fun for co-ordination.

We begin by standing up and then bend forwards and place our hands on the floor in front of us. Now try making your same hand and same leg move together, and then do the other leg and hand. It feels really fun and quite strange.

Boat (Paripurna Navasana)

Reduces fat around the waistline and tones the kidneys. In a row children can look like a Viking longboat. (Modify with bent knees.)

Sitting with our legs out in front of us and feeling our sitting bones underneath us, we hug our knees in towards our tummy. We keep our back really strong and imagine we have a shiny star on our chest, which must always be seen. Breathe in and, as we breathe out, we slowly stretch our feet towards the ceiling so that we make a V or boat shape. Try to keep your legs, knees and ankles together, and, if you feel very strong, make your legs go straight, otherwise bend your knees, which makes it a bit easier.

Stretch your arms now so that they are reaching towards your feet.

Bow (Dhanurasana)

Brings flexibility to the spine and strengthens abdominal organs, also known as a giants bowl, nest, or floating leaf.

Lying on our tummies, we bend our knees and catch our feet with our hands (or hold on to our shins). Breathe in, and, when we are ready to breathe out, we lift our feet up towards the ceiling and our chest up away from the floor. Don't forget to breathe.

Bridge (Purvottonanasana)

Strengthens wrists and ankles and expands the chest fully. A suitable pose to do after forward-bending postures. Can be a slide, bridge to a boat or castle. (Modify with knees bent.)

Sitting on our bottoms, we place our hands just behind us and make sure that our fingers are pointing forward.

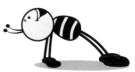

Now press down into your hands and your feet and lift your bottom off the floor and lift your tummy up towards the ceiling. If this feels a bit strong, then bend your knees and make yourself more into a table shape.

Bumpy Truck
Strengthen core stabilising muscles.

Sitting on our bottom with our legs stretched out in front of us, we sit up really tall in our back and then imagine we are holding on to a big steering wheel. As we drive we wiggle forward on our bottoms and the same sort of thing happens when we go into reverse. Hold on to your trousers, as they can drive off without you!

Butterfly (Baddha Konasana)
Helps maintain healthy function of kidneys and bladder. Can be helpful for urinary-tract infection.

Sitting up really tall on our bottoms, we bend our knees and bring the bottoms of our feet to touch. We create very gentle movement in our legs like a butterfly moving its wings in the cool summer breeze.

Cactus
A spiky balancing pose to improve concentration and focus the mind.

Standing on both feet, we look ahead and press down into one leg as we lift the other off the floor and make branch-like shapes with our arms and a pointy expression on our face.

Camel (Ustrasana)
The whole spine is stretched and the back muscles are toned. 1. hands to thigh; 2. toes tucked under and hands to heals; 3. toes extend away and hands to heals. Counterpose with Mouse. (Modify by curling toes underneath.)

We sit on our heels and then come up on to our knees. Let's try to make sure that our hips are straight over our knees and curl our toes underneath to make us feel safer. Now we place our hands just above our bottom and press into this bony area with our thumbs.

Now breathe in and, on the out breath, tuck your chin towards your chest and arch backwards. Stay for a few breaths and then come up slowly by lowering your bottom on to your heels and coming back to where you started.

Camels often travel together in camel trains, so we may need to do a few more. When we feel very comfortable in this posture, we can try to take our hands back on to our heels.

Candle (Sarvangasana)

Each child will achieve their own variation and will be able to support their body from about age four onwards by lifting their hips up and supporting their pelvis. The pose brings about a harmony and a sense of balance in the human system. The posture helps children with diges- tive disorders, poor sleeping patterns and concentration issues. (Always remember to blow out candle – nice to use if it's someone's birthday.)

Castle (see House)

Strengthens the upper arms, reduces stiffness in the shoulders and tones leg muscles.

First, let us stand with our feet wide apart so that, when we stretch our arms, our wrists are in line with our ankles. Now we take a deep breath in and, as we breathe out, we stretch our arms to the ceiling and press the palms of our hands together. Make space between our ears and our shoul- ders and be tall and pointed.

Cat (Marjariasana) variations and balance

Strengthens core stabilising muscles of abdomen and lower back.

Let's begin on all fours with our hands under our shoulders and our knees under our hips. We breathe in and push our shoulders up to the ceiling and pull our tummy up towards our back and tuck our chin in towards our chest.

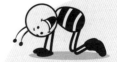

Now breathe out, and let's come back to where we started as a very brave cat.

Chair (Utkatasana)

Releases stiffness in the shoulders, strengthens the thighs evenly, tones back and abdominal muscles and fully expands the chest. Could also be Parachute.

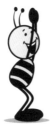

This is a strong posture for our legs which will help us to ride our bikes better and scooter and run even faster. Bring our feet about the same distance apart as our shoulders and hips. Breathe in and, as we breathe out, stretch our straight arms up to the ceiling and pretend we are going to sit down on a chair. Don't let our knees knock together and feel that our legs and backs are very strong.

Cobra (Bhujangasana)

Tones the spine and strengthens abdominal area. Also can be a child looking in a shop window, or into the witch's house, or out of a spaceship! It can be transformed into a Sphinx by bringing the elbows under the shoulders and keeping the forearms on the floor..

We lie on our tummy with our toes stretching away from us. We place our hands underneath our shoulders while tucking our elbows in close beside us. We press our pretend tail down into the floor and we push down into our hands. As we breathe out we lift our chest up away from the floor and keep our elbows tucked in and our shoulders down away from our ears.

Cow Head (Gomukhasana)

Helps to release stiffness in the hips and expand the chest. Could also be a Cow Bell.

We sit with our legs out in front of us and then bend our knees and take our feet to one side. Now, we take the top leg over the bottom so that we are sitting between both our feet, now with one knee on top of the other. This may be enough for some of us, but others might now like to take it a bit further. What we do now is take the arm on the side of the top leg behind our back and we meet it with the other arm, which reaches back over our shoulder to meet it.

That is a pretty complicated move! Now we have to repeat it on the other side!

Crab

Remember to move sideways only. Can also be Table or Table Mountain.

Sit on your bottom with your legs straight out in front of you. Now place your hands just behind your hips with your fingers facing forward. Breathe in and, on the out breath, bend your knees and press down into the feet as you lift your hips off the floor as high as you can. We can keep our head up or let it relax back if we like.

Crocodile (Chaturanga Dandasana)

In its true pose this is immensely strength-ening for wrists, torso and legs. In a more YogaBugs sense it strengthens the upper back and arms.

Chaturanga Dandasana is really for the bigger children and needs lots of strength to do. We'll stick with the YogaBugs version, which we do by lying on our side with our arms stretched out above our heads and one leg on top of the other. We snap our hands together to make big crocodile jaws and then we roll over and do them lying on our other side to catch anything that we might have missed.

Crooked Branch (Jathara Parivatanasana)

Ideal counterpose to back arches, massages abdominal organs and releases stiffness in the lower back.

We start this posture by lying on our back and hugging our knees in towards us. Now we stretch our arms out in line with our shoulders. We take a big breath in and, as we breathe out, we take both knees over to one side and we turn to look over the other shoulder. When we have done one side, we repeat and do our Crooked Branch on the other side.

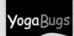
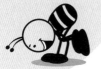

Crow (Kakasana)
Good for weak wrists and excellent for balance.

This is a posture that needs lots of balance and concentration. We start in a squatting position and place our hands just in front of us. Now we gently lean forward into our hands and keep looking ahead while we place one leg, then the other, on the backs of our arms and transfer our weight from our feet into our hands. Keep looking ahead of you at all times.

Crow Walking
Very strengthening for thigh and calf muscles, good for co-ordination in terms of linking left and right brain function.

We look very funny doing this and it is often our way of getting through the sticky mud. We start with one knee on the floor and the other knee bent with the foot on the floor. Now we have to take the opposite elbow to the knee that has the foot on the floor! If we can get that right, let's get marching through the mud or deep sand.

Cycling
Excellent for co-ordination, as above, and toning for abdominal muscles.

We lie on our backs for this one and put our hands behind our heads. We bend our knees and take one elbow towards the other knee and repeat on the other side. Remember that we do this slowly to go up the hills and very fast to come down them. We can hold our elbow to our knee when we go around a corner.

Dancer (Natarajasana)
Vertebral joints maintain their mobility and the posture is excellent for balance and in establishing poise. Recently, Dancer has been a yoga superhero. Could also be a Giant's Teapot or a Watering Can.

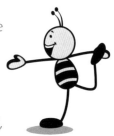

Standing on both feet and very tall, we bend one leg and raise the other arm. Now we take a breath in and, as we breathe out, we reach slightly forward with the arm and lift the leg away from us. Remember to press strongly down into our big toe on the standing foot so that we don't wobble, and then – to make sure we have really got it right – let's repeat it on the other leg.

Deer (Marichyasana)
Improves circulation to the abdominal area and mobility in the spine.

Let's start this posture by sitting up straight with our legs out in front of us. Now we bend one knee and bring the foot right up towards us. We take the arm now on the other side as the leg and push our elbow against our bent knee as we turn away from the leg and look over our shoulder with a rather superior expression on our face (like a mouse sniffing a bit of smelly cheese)! Remember that the deer always turns her head away the other way (so we do the same now with the other leg).

Diamond (preparation for Turtle/Tortoise)
Tones the spine, quietens the mind and gives an overall feeling of wellbeing and calm. (For Turtle/Tortoise, see Page 159.)

Let's sit on our bottom and bend our knees out to the side so that the bottoms of our feet are touching and making a diamond shape. Now we lean forward and take our head down towards our feet if we want to feel the posture in our hips.

Dinosaur
Good for lower back – and great fun!

We stand with our feet wide apart and our toes pointing forward. Now we take hold of our ankles and make big stomping dinosaur sounds with our feet.

Dog (Adho Mukha Svanasana)
This releases stiffness in the shoulder joints and slows the heart rate. It rejuvenates the brain cells and invigorates the brain by relieving fatigue. (This pose can also be Wolf, Hyena, Fox or Mountain.) Lamppost dog: side lift of leg on each side!

This pose can be approached lying on our tummy and putting our hands under our shoulders and then pressing down into the floor and curling our toes underneath us so that we lift up into an upside-down shape.

Otherwise we can start this posture from all fours. Remember that we press firmly down into all our fingers and keep our arms strong and our shoulders away from our ears. We push our heels down to the floor and we remember to keep lifting our bottoms towards the ceiling and keep our arms and legs strong. Our neck is soft all the time and we look back between our ankles.

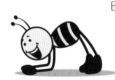

If we choose to do Lamppost Dog, then we take the weight on to one leg and lift the other up and bend our knee as a male dog might do against a lamppost. We must always remember to do both legs, as balanced yogi dogs would!

Dolphin
Strengthens the upper arm muscles and releases tightness in the shoulders (can be modified with bent knees).

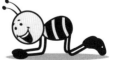

Bigger children might like to try the full posture, but let's start with the easier version. We begin on all fours and then bend our elbows and bring them to the floor. We interlace our fingers and take a breath in; we prepare to do a gentle dive forward towards our hands and, as we breathe out, we lower our body down to the floor. We breathe in and come up and repeat as many times as we feel a dolphin might dive through the waves.

If you are bigger you might like to try the same hand and elbow position but have your bottom in the air and your legs straight, as you would in dog pose. The same breathing happens as you breathe out to bring your body down to the floor and breathe in to lift up (you will feel it in your arms more like this).

Donkey Kicks
Good preparation for Handstand with older children.

We need to make sure that we have room behind us for this one and then place our hands on the floor, look ahead and then just try simple little kicks up with one leg, and then try the other. Let's not try to be too brave to start off. Let's just get the feeling first!

Dragonfly (Salabhasana)
Improves digestion and symptoms relating to it! The work on the spine is therapeutic strengthening the sacral and lumbar regions. Could also be a Cricket or a Locust.

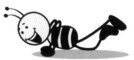

We lie on our tummy for this posture and lift one leg up in the air and then take the other leg and rest the foot on the other knee. Our hands, meanwhile, are placed under our shoulders like an insect on a branch.

Eagle (Garudasana)
Improves circulation in the hips and strengthens the legs and ankles. Can also be a knot in the elephant's trunk!

This is a great posture for gaining our balance as well as becoming strong. Let's stand with our feet together and bend our knees. Now we wrap one leg over the top of the other. If we are new to being an Eagle, we can now bring our hands to the prayer position in front of our chest and keep looking ahead. If we have done this posture a few times we can bring the elbows together and stretch the arms out. The elbow that is on the top is the one on the same side as the standing leg! Just when you think you have got it, you then do the same the other way around.

Elephants

Helps co-ordination and is a fun group activity. Children form a line, all bend forward and put their right hand between their knees and the person behind takes hold with their left hand. They then forward-march with big elephant strides and appropriate noises. (Jungle Book variation is always rather fun!)

Elephants need friends, so one of us stands in front and puts one hand through our legs and lets the other hang like a trunk. The grown-up or child stands behind and holds the arm in front of them and puts their hand through their legs – there may be others who want to join us, too. Remember that elephants hold one another's tail when they march, so don't go too fast!

Fish (Matsyasana)

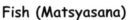

Expands the chest and helps to extend the dorsal region.

We start on our back when we are going to be fish. Now we bring our hands up alongside our tummy and bend our elbows so that we lift our head off the floor and move the chest towards the ceiling. It feels really nice in our shoulders when we do this and, while we think about, let's open and close our mouth as a fish would.

Fishing Rod (from Rowing)

Improves lymphatic functions and helps circulation in the abdominal region. Could also be a Telescope or Releasing the Sails on a Boat.

Sitting on our bottom, we bring one leg in towards us and squeeze our knee and then catch hold of that foot. Now let us see if we can reach down towards our foot on our straight leg with the other hand. YogaBugs are very good at fishing and we can do it just as well on both sides.

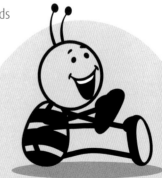

Foot Exercises (knitting feet)

Releases stiffness in the feet and can act as a 'head, neck and shoulder massage' when done correctly.

We bring our feet together as we did in the Diamond posture and Butterfly, and then interlace the toes. Sometimes it can feel a bit sore, but it certainly feels good afterwards!

Frog

Strengthens the leg and thigh muscles (see also Monkey).

This is just a mini-version of our friendly Monkey. The difference is that we do big jumps with our hands and feet on the floor from a squat position. Let's do it a few times.

Gate (Parighasana)

Helps prevent stiffness in the spine and maintains correct function of the abdominal organs. We open and close the Gate to demonstrate both sides of this posture.

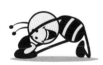

We begin on our knees and then stretch one leg out to the side, making sure that our toes point to the ceiling. We breathe in and, when we breathe out, we stretch our other arm over our head towards our stretched-out leg and enjoy a lovely long feeling down the side of our body. YogaBugs are very good with gates because we always make sure that we close them behind us (so we repeat the posture, but with the other leg).

Giraffe

Walking tall and nibbling branches with arms reaching up and both hands acting like a mouth. Just fun and interesting to watch the varying adaptations!

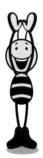

Some of us like to be giraffes by walking on our tiptoes while we stretch up and nibble the branches with our fingers. Others like to lift their long giraffe legs and continue to nibble the high branches.

Gorilla Tapping Ground (Prasarita Padottanasana)

Extends the hamstrings and reduces tightness in the lumbar spine. Gorilla can also thump chest.

We take our legs wide apart and keep our toes facing forward, and then we lean forward and tap the ground like a gorilla. When we stand up we can thump our chest, too.

Group Abdominal Breathing

A fun way of understanding abdominal breathing together. One child puts their head on another's belly and the same format continues for all. It creates a lovely laughter between everyone too.

Half-Handstand (Urdhva Muka Vrksasana)

A variation of this pose with back to the wall, hands on the floor and legs walking up the wall to a right angle. Helps to strengthen the upper body and arms while releasing tension in the neck and shoulder regions. Could also be Spider-Man Wall Walk.

This is best done when we feel quite strong in our wrists and our arms. We start by facing the wall and stretching our arms out to touch it. Now we turn around so that our back is to the wall. Place our hands on the floor and slowly walk our feet up the wall to make a table shape.

Hare

Good release in the shoulders and restful in the lower back area.

This position starts in the same way as Mouse, with our bottom back on our heels, our arms by our sides and our forehead down on the floor. Now we interlace our fingers behind our back and bring our arms over towards the floor in front of us (like the ears on a hare).

Hero (Virasana)

Excellent work on the inward rotation of the hip joints, improves circulation in the legs and can be restful after a lot of activity.
Could also be a Thai Goddess.

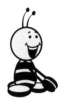

We begin on our knees and then pull the muscles of our lower legs out to the side so that our feet point backward and our knees are together. If we feel comfy like this and we can keep our knees together, we can lie down on the floor and be a resting hero.

Horse

Good extension in the hip flexors, which can in turn improve back arching postures. (This can also be Unicorn or Zebra.)

We can start this posture on our knees and then step one foot forward as far as it feels comfortable. We now stretch forward and can bring our arms up in front of us and press our hands together as our ears or as a unicorn.

Hot-Air Balloon

Using inhalation through the nose and exhalation through the mouth while taking the arms in a circle above the head.

This posture helps to make us feel calm because we often close our eyes when we do it and we imagine the huge colourful hot-air balloon filling up above us. It is nice to start by making a circle with the hands by touching the fingertips together. As we breathe in and out the balloon gets bigger and the arms reach up to make a circle with the fingers touching above our head.

House (see Castle)
Good for extension in the arms and strengthening in the legs.

Can also be Rocket, Eiffel Tower or a Pyramid or Tent.

We stand with our feet wide apart so that, when we stretch our arms, our wrists are in line with our ankles. Now we take in a deep breath and, as we breathe out, we stretch our arms to the ceiling and press the palms of our hands together. We make space between our ears and our shoulders and stand tall and pointed.

Hugs
Can be very helpful in releasing tension in the rhomboid muscles under the shoulder blades and can be useful in stimulating the back of the lungs. Cross the arms and take the fingers to the back to touch the shoulder blades. (See Baby Bird.)

We all know how to do these, and we just have to remember to use one arm on top and then the other, because we can never just give one hug!

Humming Breath (Brahmari)
Very calming to the mind and helpful for withdrawal of the senses. Can be a bumble bee.

This is very calming and helps us to find a still place inside us. We put our fingers softly in our ears and breathe in through our nose and then make a humming sound as we breathe out.

Leg Raises (Supta Padangustasana)
Improves stiffness in the hips and back of the legs. (Can be Moon Walking Sleepwalking or Spiderman.)

This posture makes our legs feel long and strong. We start doing this one on our backs. We take a big breath in through our nose and lift one leg (keeping it as straight as we can) towards the ceiling. As we breathe out we lower it to the floor and repeat on the other side.

Imagine walking on a ceiling like this or having special powers to help you walk up walls or through the clouds.

Lightning (Standing Twist)

Tones abdominal muscles and maintains flexibility in the spine.

This can be done like a Crooked Branch (see Page 141) or alternatively we can stand with our feet together and swing our body round one way and then back the other way. Let's make sure that our arms are straight like great flashes of lightning through the sky.

Lion (Simhasana)

A great stress buster and the children love it. (Can also be Tiger.)

We all love this posture because it gets rid of any difficult feelings or thoughts that might be annoying us. We sit back on our heels, close our eyes, count to three and come up on to our knees. We take a deep breath in and, as we breathe out, we open our eyes, open our mouth, stick out our tongue and make an aaaaahhh sound to scare away any grown-ups.

Lotus flower opening and closing

Strengthens abdominal muscles and lengthens hamstrings. Can also be done with backs to centre and legs out like an octopus. Start in paschimottanasana (see Pizza on Page 154), then to dandasana (see preparation for sandwich on Page 156) and then stretch arms up like the stamen.

This combination of postures is great for making our legs feel stretchy and our bodies relaxed. We start in Sandwich (see Page 156) and then we sit up on our bottoms with our backs straight (like the lotus flower opening to the sun). We stretch our arms up so that we attract bugs and bees to our beautiful flower. From sitting we come forward again into sandwich.

We then roll back to sitting and come forward again into Sandwich as the sun sets and we close our lotus flowers for the night.

Magic Bird

Helpful for lengthening hamstrings, releasing stiffness in the shoulders and a powerful breathing exercise.

This posture is lovely for imagining how wonderful it must feel to fly. We stand with our feet together and we bend forward so that our body is in a straight line so that we bend only halfway to the floor.

We stretch our arms out to the side as we breathe in and when we breathe out we bring our hands to meet in the middle. We repeat this as a Magic Bird would when it flies us off on mystical adventures.

Mermaid (Bharadvajasana)

An easy and uncomplicated twist for children and helpful for stiff lumbar and dorsal spines.

We sit on our bottom and take our legs over to one side. We make a little saucer shape with our foot underneath and then rest the top foot in it. Keeping our knees together, we twist away from our bent knees to look over our shoulder. This posture is for mermaids or mermen and needs to be done on both sides.

Monkey

Similar to frog but with higher jumps.

This posture is like doing great big star jumps. We squat down on our heels and then jump up super-high while making monkey-like sounds!

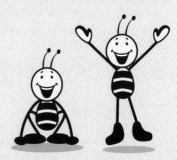

Mouse (Balasana)

A quiet pose where the forehead rests on the floor and helps to focus the mind. An excellent counterpose to the Dog posture and very good after back arches (Can also be Rock, Cloud or Hiding Place, Hedgehog.)

This is a lovely resting pose. We sit back on our heels and rest our arms by our side and our forehead on the floor. We relax our shoulders which helps us to feel still and quiet.

Mountain (Tadasana)

All the ingredients for good posture and gait.

This helps us to feel tall and balanced. It is very good to see if we can keep our ears over our shoulders, our shoulders over our hips, our hips over our knees and our knees over our ankles. Our feet are together and we stand as tall as we can with our neck feeling long and our face relaxed.

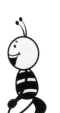

Owl

From kneeling: good arm extension and helps maintain flexibility in the toes.

We sit back on our heels with our toes curled underneath us. As we breathe in we raise our arms up over our head (like huge owl wings) and we come up on to our knees. When we breathe out we lower our bottom back on to our heels and our arms come down to our sides again.

Oysters

Hip opener and forward bend. Children sit with the soles of their feet together with fingers interlaced held above their heads (like the top of the shell) and take the feet a little further away from their bodies. They come into a forward bend over their feet.

This posture starts from Butterfly (see Page 138), and then we fold forward to take our head down towards the floor so that we can close our shells and feel very private, as oysters do.

Penguin

Charlie Chaplin-style walk – great fun and very silly.

We stand with our feet together and then turn our toes out to the sides. Now we walk, pressing down into the front of our feet and lowering into our heels. Remember to wiggle and wobble like a penguin.

Pigeon (Eka Pada Rajakapotasana)
Maintains mobility in the hips and flexibility in the lower back.

This posture is best done from the Dog pose (see Page 143). We bend one knee and bring it forward while we stretch the back leg away on the floor. We try to make both hips feel level and we bring the toes on the bent leg underneath the hip on the other leg. We should feel a bit of work in our hips now. This is called King Pigeon pose, so we can bring our hands together on our chest in prayer position and then bend forward like a bow and stretch our arm out along the floor in front of us. Remember that we must do the same on the other side and show how good we are at doing it with both our legs.

Pizza (Paschimottanasana)
Improves digestive and kidney functions, maintains flexibility in the spine and is restful for the mind. (See Sandwich on Page 156.)

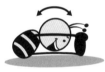

Plank
Excellent for the core stabilising muscles of the abdomen and lower back.

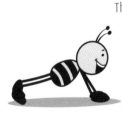

This is a very strong posture, which also makes us feel really strong. We start on all fours and then stretch our legs out straight so that we feel the weight between our hands and our feet with our toes curled underneath us. We feel our tummies and our legs working very hard, and our wrists and arms get stronger too.

Playing the Piano
Keeps fingers supple. Encourage children to play an 'air' piano.

This is lovely for making all our fingers work, so we imagine that we are playing on a huge piano and that we are the best pianists in the world.

Princess

Good for proprioceptive (nerve-end) feedback from muscles and joints. Children walk on their tiptoes with an air of dignity and elegance!

This is fun for making our feet work well and to stop our toes from getting stiff. We simply walk about and stay on tiptoes all the time. Careful not to wobble too much!

Rabbit

Good action in the legs, hip opener and fun to do. Place hands on the floor in a deep squat. Move hands forward and jump feet up to meet the hands moving forward rabbit style!

We start this posture from a squat and take our arms forward so that our legs then follow, and we jump them to the outside of our hands as rabbits do.

Rag Doll

Uttanasana: helps to ease stomach pains and calms a busy mind. Strengthens the legs.

We stand with our legs together or a bit wider if we feel more comfortable, and then we fold forward, hands down, letting our arms and shoulders feel completely relaxed.

Roadrunner

Lengthens the hip flexors. Lunge as in sun sequence with palms of hands on floor.

We use this posture when we are doing our Sun Salutation (see Page 135). One foot is forward and the other leg stretches back – the way runners do just before they start a race. We have our hands on the floor either side of our bent knees and we can make a Road Runner beep-beep sound, before swapping to the other leg and doing the same again.

Rowing

Releases stiffness in the hips, can be made
stronger by answering the phone (foot to ear) or
striking a match, or developed into rocking a baby
with the foot in the opposite elbow. Ensure that the
heel follows the line of the opposite leg.

Sitting up nice and tall with our legs in front of us, we reach down and take the toes of one foot and hold it with both hands. As we breathe in, we bend the knee and bring the foot all the way up the other leg and, as we breathe out, we take it all the way down it again. Our knee comes out to the side as we do this so that we feel as if we are massaging our hips.

Remember that we go in circles if we don't practise on both legs. Often the phone rings when we are rowing and we have to take our foot to our ear. Alternatively, the baby cries and we have to rock them back to sleep. There are always two phone calls and twins, so we get to do both legs!

Sandwich (Paschimottanasana)

The benefits are the same as for Pizza, above (see Page 154). Could also be packing a suitcase. Good preparation for packing a suitcase is to reach up to the top shelf with stretched-out arms to get it down. This posture is also good for spreading butter and cheese and chopping ingredients.

We sit with our legs out in front of us and we spread the butter all over the bottom of our sandwich (or the cheese on our pizza) and then we fill them with delicious goodies from our toes to our thighs. We lean forward and gobble everything up as quickly as possible so that no one else can get there before us.

Shark

Based on Snake (below), but interlace the fingers behind
the back and roll from side to side. Can also be Superhero by taking arms alongside the body.

Let's start this posture lying on our tummy and then
we interlace our fingers behind our back like a shark
fin. YogaBugs sharks are kind and always promise
that they won't eat us, so we just practise rolling gently from side to side as we move through the water.

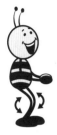

Skiing

Strengthens the knees and improves mobility in the hips. Stand in tadasana (see Mountain on Page 153), bend the knees and move the hips slalom style.

With our feet together we swing our hips from side to side as cool skiers do.

Sphinx (see Cobra)

Spider Stretch

Exercises the legs and tones the lumbar and coccyx regions of the spine.

We take our feet wide apart and then hold on to our heels with our hands. When we feel strong and ready, we start to straighten our long spider legs.

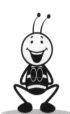

Squats (Malasana)

Tones the abdominal organs and relieves lower-back stiffness.

Some grown-ups can't do this at all, but when we are smaller we find it easier. We simply sit back on our heels with our knees bent and our arms stretched out in front of us.

Star

Releases stiffness in the shoulders, encourages length in the spine and opens the hip area. See Oysters (Page 153), but have hands in the prayer position on the top of the head.

Stork/Flamingo

Good for concentration and balance and strengthening in the standing leg.

Standing on both legs, we then bend one so that our foot is touching our bottom and we hold on to it with our hand. With the other hand we stretch up to the ceiling and look straight ahead while we wait for our fish.

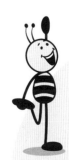

Sun Circle (Upavista Konasana)

Stretches hamstrings and helps blood to circulate correctly in the pelvic region. Look into rock pool or down at Earth. Can also be a magic carpet with sideways, forward and backward movements.

We need a few friends for this one. We sit in a big circle with all our legs stretched out wide. We can lean over one way and then the other and then stretch forward into the middle of the circle.

Surfing (Virabhadrasana 2)

Tones the abdominal area, tones and strengthens the calves and thighs.

Step the feet wide apart so that the wrists are above the ankles. Turn one foot out and the back foot slightly in. Breathe in and when we breathe out we stretch the arms as wide as possible to the side and we bend our front knee. Now we look down the arm over the bent knee and think what cool surfers we are.

Tent (Prasarita Padotanasana)

As per Gorilla Tapping Ground (Presarita Padotanasana), but arms are straight from floor. Can also be the entrance to a cave.

We take our feet wide apart and then lean forward, bending our knees if we need to so that we can bring our hands under our shoulders on the floor. Younger members of the family might like to crawl through the door and into the tent.

Thunder

A loud clap above the head is just fun.

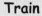

Train

Good for co-ordination and working together as a group. Helps to integrate left and right brain function through cross-body action of arms and legs.

We stand at the front and others, including grown-ups, stand behind. We imagine that we are a train slowly leaving the station so we start gently raising one arm and the other leg and then get gradually faster as we are followed down the track.

Tree (Vrksana)

Strengthens the ankles and legs, relieves lower-back stiffness.

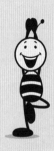

Standing on both legs we bend one, while keeping the other really strong. We place our foot on our ankle, our lower leg or the top of our thigh. Sometimes we have good balancing days and on others it feels really windy and our trees don't balance so well. Remember that we must always try it on both legs.

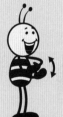

Tumble Dryer

Helps focus on breath and quietens the mind.

We bring our fingers together in line with our mouth and then we breathe in through our nose and out softly through our mouth, like a soft silent whistle.

Turtle/Tortoise (Kurmasana)

Excellent benefits by stilling the senses and increasing energy levels. Children are often very good at this – rather better than their parents!

See Diamond (Page 143), and from this posture we take our arms underneath our knees and behind us so that we try to touch our fingers behind our backs.

Volcano
Good breathing exercise. Can also be swimming up from underwater or swimming to the surface after a dive.

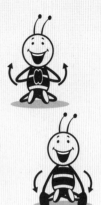

We start in the Mountain pose (see Page 153) and bring our hands on to our chest in the prayer position. We breathe in and stretch both our hands to the ceiling and, as we breathe out, we take our arms back down to our sides. We repeat this a few times as it helps us to feel calm.

Washing Machine
Opens the hips and releases tightness in the shoulders.

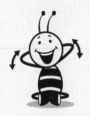

Sitting cross-legged, we put our hands behind our head and we breathe in and then breathe out and twist one way, breathe in and come back to the middle, and breathe out to turn the other way. Remember that we can speed up the machine so that it really washes our clothes well.

Whale (Sethu Bandha)
Maintains mobility in the lower back, strengthens legs and knees and releases tightness in the neck and shoulders (we play Bubble Pop by chanting as below).

We start this posture lying on our back and bending our heels in so that they are in line with our sitting bones and hip width apart. We try to feel as if our lower back is touching the floor and then we breathe in and lift our hips and our back off the floor and move our chest towards our chin. We do this saying, 'Bubble, bubble, bubble' and we pop when we blow out the water through our tummy button, which is our whale blowhole. It is fun to repeat this a few times until we get all the bubbles and pops in the right order.

Windmill

Excellent for releasing tightness in the arms and shoulders and excellent counterpose to back arches.

We step our feet wide apart and take one arm across our body to the other leg. Then we turn and look up at the other arm, which is stretching up to the ceiling. We breathe in and, when we breathe out, we swap to the other side.

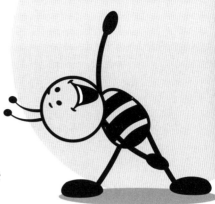

Woodchopper

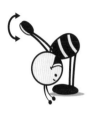

Removes stiffness in the shoulders and strengthens the legs.

Let's step our feet wide apart and join our hands behind our backs. As we breathe in we lift our chest to the ceiling and when we breathe out we bring our hands over our head towards the floor.

Chapter 8
Visualisation and Affirmations

POSITIVE VISUALISATION: WHY DO IT, AND HOW TO MAKE IT FUN!

The magical powers of a child's imagination will fascinate you. Rudolph Steiner (anthroposophist and founder of the Steiner Schooling System) believed that children don't really 'come in to land' in the world until their first teeth fall out. A child's imaginative powers are very real to them and their true belief that they are the creature or animal in the story is enchanting. Sharing this magical time with them through yoga, relaxation and visualisation creates a very special experience.

Visualisation techniques are woven into the relaxation time at the end of the YogaBugs session. Guided imagery helps to tap into rich visual images that can help children to relax into learning while acquiring better listening skills, improving their creative ability and developing better artistic, academic and sporting ability. Children become more aware of each other's feelings and are naturally more sensitive in their behaviour. Working together with children through visualisation helps to create a feeling of inner calm and harmony.

Libby Hartman, director of the Chelsea Group of Children, says, 'Many children have weakness in creating mental images, which causes difficulty in reading and oral comprehension. Combining yoga with a story means that children are able to visualise.' She goes on to explain, 'When a child participates in creating a sequence of events or becomes the description of an object or animal, the words turn into richly detailed sensory images. By stimulating visualisation we help children improve their expressive and receptive language skills.'

Guided imagery acts as a tool to release creativity and, the more consistent we are in working with visualisation techniques, the more successful the results. Don't have high expectations in the first few sessions, because it takes you and your child time to settle into the routine, and wriggling, giggling and wanting to chat are perfectly normal. It is helpful to dim the lights, ensure that you and your child are warm and comfortable and use the relaxation techniques to encourage a more peaceful state.

Visualisation helps children to be present in the moment rather than thinking about what might be happening next. It allows time for reflection as opposed to meeting the regular deadlines of their daily little lives.

Young children often learn through their senses, remembering objects around them, the smell of cooking, the feeling of rocking to get a rhythm for learning times tables etc. We all have the potential to find our creativity and it is through imagery that we are able to take off the outer leaves and find the succulent centre – the intelligence in ourselves. We all enjoy daydreaming, and visualisation is very much along the same lines.

Our goal in doing visualisation with our child is simply to decrease stress, boost learning and develop memory. There is so little time in our lives to reflect and be in the present moment. Teaching our children to relax and enjoy visualisation techniques may prove to be a most valuable gift.

As with relaxation techniques, visualisation can be used on journeys and to help children feel more positive about themselves when life sometimes gets too much for them.

POSITIVE AFFIRMATIONS NURTURE INHERENT CONFIDENCE

Affirmations are important tools that can help to bring about change. They can also be very powerful in improving a child's view of themselves and their abilities. They can affect change physically, mentally and emotionally if practised with confidence.

It is helpful to finish your session together with a positive affirmation. This helps us to feel better and able to reach the goals that we strive for in life. This might be as simple as getting all your spellings right, or winning a race, or eating all your greens.

Affirmations make us feel better and more positive, and help us to ride the waves in life. They take our minds to the place where we feel happy about ourselves and give us the focus we need for what is good in our lives. Children respond well to positive affirmations, because the very young are still undeniably connected to the strength of their inner self. If we as adults can guide children into believing in their own ability, we hope that we can build a more confident generation.

In our lives today, we do not seem to spend enough time valuing who and what we are. Through constructive affirmation, we can help to develop a strong relationship with our children that could help them to maintain confidence in themselves. At the same time we are, as parents, relations and friends, helping to understand the power of the word and the strength of affirmations, which may in turn help us to communicate better with our children.

How often do we hear ourselves repeating what our parents said to us? Is it constructive and is it helping our children to grow positively in their thinking and creating? Recognise the regret we feel when we insult our children or say things that we do not mean afterwards. I love it when I tell small children how clever they are, how fast they run, how well they sing or how pretty or handsome they are, and they respond by saying, 'I know!' However, I do not think we should make quite such a high value of ourselves public! I do feel that we can help children to maintain their self-esteem by feeling it inside, through positive praise. Happy, positive children grow into successful, fulfilled adults. Comments that honour a child's behaviour are internalised and nurtured; such remarks will help them to share love, praise and respect.

We can stimulate positive thinking and encourage our children to develop into confident and happy individuals.

The time when children are most receptive to positive affirmations is during their final relaxation, visualisation or at the end of the class.

Here are some simple and uncomplicated affirmations:

* I feel still and happy.
* I feel at peace.
* I am strong and I will do well.
* I would like to be able to be kind and to forgive.
* I am happy as me.
* I feel a big smile inside.
* I feel a warm sun shining inside me.
* I am the best me I could possibly be.
* I am a good person.
* I am relaxed.
* I feel happy and beautiful/handsome.

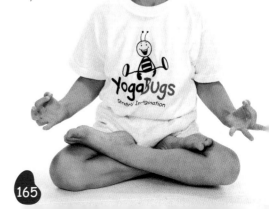

Chapter 9
Yoga Principles in YogaBugs

YogaBugs incorporates the elements of hatha yoga, using breathing, posture and relaxation/visualisation techniques, and is designed to appeal to children. Hatha yoga is based on a system of eight limbs or steps, which were devised by the ancient Indian sage Patanjali. These 'codes of conduct' can be made child-friendly and incorporated or themed into adventures.

Many of these elements are taught throughout a YogaBugs adventure in a way that appeals to the age group. When introducing yoga to children, it is valuable to uphold these principles to encourage the children to live with awareness and respect.

Patanjali's Yoga Sutras are eight principles that form the foundation of all yoga instruction and practice. They are integral to all aspects of yoga and lead to a better quality of life. Children will enjoy finding their own examples and including them in their practice. As the children gain in confidence, and understand more about yoga and how it works, they may like to create their own stories around the various limbs of yoga.

So many of us think that yoga is just a physical practice. Patanjali inspires us all with his knowledge and valuable advice, even thousands of years later. When I first encountered Patanjali, I found it hard to believe that such ancient wisdom could still apply to our lives, but how wrong I was!

PATANJALI'S EIGHT PRINCIPLES

1. Yamas
These are moral principles based on the following.

* Non-violence (*ahimsa*), which includes things that we want but that may not be good for us or may not be things

that we need. It also means avoiding unnecessary attacks on brothers, sisters and friends or having self-defeating thoughts.

* Truth and honesty (*satya*) and telling no lies. It is valuable to give children time to reflect on telling the truth and how important it is to be true to ourselves so we can be true to others.

* Non-stealing (*asteya*) material things such as toys, as well as attention away from our friends or family.

* Non-lust (*bramacharya*), which in essence means self-discipline, making sure that you help children to understand simple routines such as always washing their hands before they eat, cleaning their teeth morning and night.

* Non-possessiveness (*aparigraha*), which is not feeling the need to surround yourself with material things such as the scooter that your friend Joey has, but instead keeping life simple and being happy with the good things that you do have.

2. Niyamas
These concern how we treat ourselves, and are based on the following.

* Purity (*shauca*), which in essence follows the principles of the five yamas above, but simply means keeping yourself, your clothes and your surroundings clean and tidy as well as understanding the values of healthy food and exercise. This can be easily identified by keeping your room neat, eating fresh fruit and vegetables and walking to school when you can.

* Contentment (*santosha*), which is finding happiness in what you have, and enjoying the moment rather than wishing for more. This is particularly true of a television programme, when children always want just five minutes more, and we're all familiar with this – especially at bedtime!

* Austerity (*tapas*), disciplining oneself to seek higher spiritual goals and achieve one's ambitions. This could be simplified into doing what you are asked when you are asked and

spending a little bit of time before sleep thinking about family and friends and people in the world who need love and support.

* Study of the sacred texts (*svadhyaya*) or reading books that inspire and teach you. For YogaBugs this could be simplified into positive affirmations that help children to feel good about themselves.

* Surrendering the ego (*Ishvar Pranidhana*). This can be made easier by saying 'yes' rather than 'no' and expressing willingness! It is also valuable to help children to understand other people's feelings by putting themselves in a similar position: how would they feel if . . .?

3. Asana
This involves postures, that is to say the actual physical work that helps to still the mind in preparation for relaxation and visualisation. They maintain flexibility, tone and strengthen the body while helping to release tension in the muscles. Posture work can also free the body from symptoms of anxiety, notably tightness in the shoulders and neck areas.

4. Pranayama
This concerns the control of the breath. Not only does correct breathing focus and purify the mind, but it also removes distractions.

5. Pratyahara
This is, quite simply, withdrawing the senses. This tends to begin during the process of relaxation, where outside distractions become less noticeable. It is the time when children are encouraged to let all the busy-ness in their minds fade, so that they can feel and sense a quietness in their head and in their body.

6. Dharana
This principle involves stilling the mind, and Patanjali says, 'Concentration is binding thought in one place.' This can be achieved by focusing the attention on a candle flame or by repeating a mantra

(such as 'I feel peaceful') or through visualisation. *Dharana* occurs when there is no sense of time or space.

7. Dhyana

This is simply the next stage on from dharana, when you are not aware of distraction. It is a complete union of mind and body – a feeling of stillness both within and around you. For children this can often be explained as being like the moment just before you fall asleep, the time when you feel warm, safe and comfortable but still just awake.

8. Samadhi

This one is really the icing on the cake! It is a state of total bliss and union with a higher self. There are some who can achieve this elevated state while on Earth! It is within all of us; it can be reached through dedication and commitment to yoga.

POSTURES FOR CHILDHOOD DIFFICULTIES

Practising yoga can have a positive effect on a number of childhood conditions, from asthma to learning difficulties. Here are some of the common conditions that can benefit from the effects of yoga, and the main postures and breathing techniques that are particularly beneficial for each.

Poor concentration

Through the posture work and, notably, balancing postures, which are woven into the adventures, children are encouraged to focus their gaze ahead of them (*drishti*).This can help to improve mental concentration.

Postures that work on lengthening the spine such as the forward- (Sandwich) and back-bending poses (Camel), activate the spine and stimulate the nervous system.

Postures where the head is below the heart too can be helpful, such as downward Dog pose, which is an inversion, since they improve

circulation of blood and oxygen to the brain and develop the concentration span.

Hyperactivity
This needs to be approached differently, for, while the symptoms are
based on poor concentration, the technique is to quieten the child
through focused breathing techniques and postures such as Sandwich and Star. These help children to draw their thoughts inwards,
because trying to think about one object or thought is challenging
for them. Sun salutations help these children as they have to think
about synchronising breath with movement.

As children get older, inversions can also be helpful, since they have
a quietening effect on the nervous system.

It will take time to see the benefits of yoga for these children, but
the combination of physical posture work and gentle relaxation can
soon start to show. Continuity is important, because children with
hyperactivity are resistant to change, so it is helpful to create a
peaceful environment from which to practise together, perhaps with
candles and appropriate music with as few distractions around them
as possible.

Headaches
Yoga postures will release tension in the neck and shoulders,
increase circulation to the head, stimulate the nervous system and
help alleviate pain. These include Candle, Dog and Crooked Branch.
Yogic breathing exercises can calm the mind, reduce stress and alleviate anxiety. Meditation reduces stress, calms the mind and reduces
negative feelings. This can be as simple as candle gazing or asking
children to repeat a simple mantra such as 'I am peace'.

Constipation and stomach ache
Deep abdominal breathing can be effective, as can rocking and rolling backwards and forwards while hugging the knees together. It is
important to encourage children to drink lots of water. In the winter
this is valuable because our houses and classrooms are hot and

centrally heated while, in the summer, hot days can also be very dehydrating.

Try back arches such as Cobra and twists such as Mermaid as well as squatting. As a parent, you may find it helpful, also, to massage gently the tummy by walking the fingers across from right to left.

Sinus problems

Sun Salutations can be effective in bringing balance to the body and clearing a blocked nose. Inversions such as Dog, the standing forward bend and Candle will also be helpful. Back arches such as Fish and Bow can help relieve symptoms of congestion.

Asthma

Simple breathing techniques, such as maintaining the inhalation and exhalation for the same duration (e.g. breathe in for a count of six, breathe out for a count of six) can be helpful. Encourage a pause between the exhalation and subsequent inhalation to build up the carbon dioxide levels in the lungs (this is the basis of the Buteyko Technique). Ideally children need to try a count of one, then inhale again. Then they count, one, two and so on until they can pause for up to ten counts prior to breathing in again.

Advise children to lie over sofa arms or bolsters to help open the congested area.

Yoga has come a long way towards healing and managing asthma, and postures that open the chest area and reduce anxiety are beneficial to children with this problem. Helpful positions are reclining Hero and reclining Butterfly. Instead of allowing the back to be on the floor, a rolled-up towel can be placed along the length of the spine and under the head. Alternatively, a pile of books (telephone directories are ideal) can be put lengthways under the shoulder blades while supporting the head. Children then relax their shoulders and release tension across the chest area.

Chapter 10
Additional Support

By introducing yoga into the lives of children who have special educational needs, you will focus their concentration, while positive reinforcement will help to build their self-esteem and confidence. Physiologically, yoga will help develop low muscle tone and reduce spasm in areas of the body with high muscle tone. It will increase a child's flexibility, which will, in turn, give children a clearer understanding of their body and how it can work for them. Children will also have a clearer understanding of where they are in space (proprioception) and of their body parts, and where they are in relation to each other.

We have outlined briefly some areas of Additional Needs and made suggestions about how to encourage children to do yoga by highlighting some of the benefits for them. Naturally we also recognise that you as the parent or carer of the child will be a great deal more knowledgeable and experienced in working with your children. However, we hope that you will still find that yoga can offer some advantages to your child or children.

LEARNING DIFFICULTIES AND LOW DEVELOP-MENTAL DELAY

Overview
Parents are frequently concerned if their child shows signs of learning issues at school. Naturally, there may be any number of reasons for not reaching age-appropriate targets in school, but often such issues relate to a particular learning difficulty.

Interestingly, children with learning issues often have a normal range of intelligence. They strive to follow instructions, to concentrate, and 'be well behaved' in their home and school environments.

However, regardless of this effort, they may not understand school assignments and as a result they do not achieve their goals. Learning difficulties can affect at least one schoolchild in ten.

A child born with a learning difficulty is not necessarily someone who cannot learn. Instead, the child may just have a processing problem, such as a visual or auditory processing impairment that makes their ability to learn from routine ways of teaching more challenging and difficult.

Research carried out by the American Academy of Child and Adolescent Psychiatry has shown that learning disabilities are triggered by a complexity in the nervous system, which processes messages relating to receiving, processing and communicating information. This can be combined with symptoms of hyperactivity which makes it difficult for these children to sit still and not be distracted.

What are these disorders and how can yoga help?

These are disorders that hinder a child's ability to read, write, communicate and perform to their age appropriate levels. Disorders that may be familiar to you are dyslexia and dyspraxia. Children with dyslexia often find difficulty in their body positioning and co-ordination, while they are also challenged in numeracy and sport skills and any task that requires sequencing.

While so many sporting activities at school have a competitive aspect to them, yoga for children with dyspraxia benefits them enormously, since it does not require the hand–eye co-ordination of ball games and other team sports. It helps children to become aware of their bodies, and they also benefit from having a spot or mat to return to, since this stops them wandering.

Yogic breathing exercises strengthen the immune system and improve the function of the central nervous system. The balancing postures develop concentration levels while the posture work helps to improve body awareness. Holding postures for a little longer helps these children to establish body awareness. The relaxation and visualisation techniques are good for concentration and memory.

Children with dyslexia benefit from clear and simple instruction. It is often helpful to start by introducing them to the Mouse pose so that they become spatially aware of their bodies and their breathing. Breathing helps these children to focus and listen.

For children with poor co-ordination issues and clumsiness it can be very helpful to take them back through the journey of development using these movements as warm-up exercises.

* Ask them to lie on their back and hold their feet in a happy-baby pose.

* Ask them to turn on to the side and then on to the tummy.

* Ask them to raise the head and upper body gradually.

* Then ask them to come to all fours, and encourage them to balance on one hand and raise the opposite leg behind them. This works on the brain in the same way as crawling does.

* Often these children will not have crawled, and this process will help integrate the left and right hemispheres of the brain, which makes new learning easier for them. Children with dyslexia have benefited from the eye exercises, which help to develop the optic nerve and in turn encourage the brain to work more effectively.

ATTENTION-DEFICIT DISORDER AND ATTENTION-DEFICIT AND HYPERACTIVITY DISORDER

Overview
The information given here is nonspecific and no one child will show the same symptoms. These children will benefit from making eye contact and will respond to hearing their name. Be prepared to give reminders to the child and to praise them for their efforts.

Attention-deficit disorder (ADD) is a continual pattern where children lack concentration and behave in a hyperactive, inattentive or day-dreamy manner relative to their level of development. You, as the adult, need to be aware of how important it is to nurture and support the child.

What is it?

ADD and attention-deficit and hyperactivity disorder (ADHD) may arise because the brain is not processing sensory information effectively, and may be due to chemical imbalances, brain damage, genetics and/or food intolerances. Staying still is almost impossible for children with these problems, and they may find it difficult to concentrate for prolonged periods.

Factors that can increase such behaviour are artificial light, especially strip lighting, television and computers, as well as crowded places, changes in temperature, strong wind and noise.

Associated behaviours include: hyperactivity, speaking or acting before thinking, difficulty in following instructions, poor organisational skills, restlessness, impatience, forgetfulness, low self-esteem, and poor social skills. Children with ADHD find it difficult to slow down, even when they want to; often they are so hurried that they seem clumsy and unco-ordinated.

How yoga can help

Once you have established a level of trust with the child, you will find that the postural, breathing and relaxation techniques of yoga work essentially on the central nervous system. The more spiritual side helps improve internal connection by focusing the mind. Yogic breathing techniques have proved very successful in calming and focusing children at the start of a story. Yoga, breathing and relaxation techniques can also be used as life skills at other times.

By developing a relationship with the child in an activity they will enjoy and benefit from, you are helping to improve their confidence, concentration and sense of wellbeing. Generally, squeezing postures (preparation for Eagle, or *garudasana*) are good for children with self-confidence issues and ADD. Children will also enjoy rolling and rocking movements. Tensing and relaxing the limbs helps to soothe the nervous system and sideways stretches help to diffuse anger as they work on the gall-bladder meridian.

Autistic-Spectrum Disorder
Overview

Children with autistic-spectrum disorder (ASD) will all present with different needs. I understand it as a developmental and communication disorder that may affect their ability to form relationships and ability to communicate effectively.

ASD can affect children in varying degrees, some quite mildly and others to a more severe degree. It is found more commonly in boys than girls and includes Asperger syndrome (see Page 180), and in turn has a suggested link to ADD and ADHD (see Page 174). For example, some children may exhibit aggressive and disruptive behaviour; others may repeat movements and communicate by gestures or sounds; some just appear to be in a world of their own. In almost all cases that I have seen, all children on the autistic spectrum have very low muscle tone and are often left-handed. The cross-mid-line challenges of postures such as cycling and climbing that YogaBugs offers can support and assist these children at many different levels. Activities that cross the mid-line help these children to integrate the functions of the left and right sides of their brain.
There are three main areas of difficulty:

* social interaction;

* social communication;

* theory of mind, i.e. the ability to understand things from a different point of view – so it is difficult for them to be a fish swimming through the ocean; these children are very visual learners so pictures are often more helpful than speech.

When giving instructions, don't reinforce them in a different way. Stay with exactly the same words, or else the child will understand it as a new instruction which produces more work for you.
These children also need routine, they do not like change.

How yoga can help

Developing your own bond with your child can come through telling them stories, sharing music and movement or playing a game and gradually introducing aspects of a story.

If you are not working with your own child, it is always important to liaise with the parents to understand the best way of working together with their child. Breathing exercises and relaxation techniques can create the foundation from which the child can grow and thrive. Once these are established, then the posture work can develop.

By bringing the focus of the mind (through correct breathing techniques) together with the movement of the body, yoga offers autistic children the opportunity to improve their mobility, memory and communication skills. Children with autism enjoy routine, familiarity and stability. Some children find it hard to imagine, so being an animal, bird, fish or tree is very hard for them. It is, in these cases, much easier to describe going in and out of the posture without identifying the animal, tree, etc. itself. Sometimes the opposite can happen and these children will totally immerse themselves in the character and will wish to be treated solely as that character such as Thomas the Tank Engine, Superman, Bratz.

Children with ASD may not understand general instructions until you say their name at the start and they realise that you are talking to them, so using their name to focus them can be very helpful. They find social communication very difficult and need rules and an understanding of the themes. You can help your child by starting each story with the same posture, because it can help them to feel more secure.

Detailed below are five examples of how autism can make you feel, by kind permission from the National Autistic Society.

1. To you, she is upset about something; to a person with autism, they don't know how she feels.

Even if you'd never met this girl, your instinct would be to ask if she is OK, to offer her some comfort. But someone with autism wouldn't know how to react, making it hard for them to respond. Not being able to interact socially with people in ways most of us take for granted can make someone with autism feel very isolated and frustrated.

2. To you, a soft, cuddly teddy; to a person with autism: 'I can't hold him because his fur hurts my hands.'

Someone with autism can be extremely sensitive to the texture and feel of things. Eating custard can be like eating sand, or the finest silk blouse can feel like wearing barbed wire. Can you imagine the frustration of not feeling comfortable in your own clothes? Even the softest human touch can feel like acute pain, making it impossible to offer a consoling hug or physical contact.

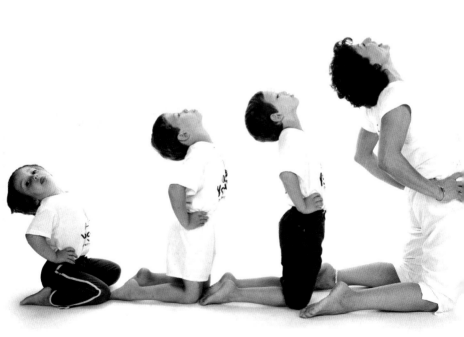

3. To you, a lovely red cake; to a person with autism: 'I can't eat it because it's got red on it.'

Imagine being terrified of the colour red: not being able to wear it, touch it or even go near it. You couldn't use a postbox, eat anything red, no matter how hungry you were. Yet the fear of particular colours is just the sort of thing someone with autism has to live with every day.

4. To you, let's play; to a person with autism: 'I can't play because there aren't any rules.'

For most kids, playtime is the highlight of the day. For children with autism, it's the time they dread most, because it means interacting with others. Play works for a child with autism only if they follow very strict rules and never break them. The frustration they feel at being excluded is matched only by the pain their parents experience, knowing their child cannot join in as they would like them to do.

5. To you we're camping; to a person with autism: 'I can see twenty-eight tents: eight blue, six yellow, five green and nine multicoloured.'

People with autism see everything at once, right down to the tiniest detail. In a new place where there is a lot to take in, this can be overwhelming, causing great anxiety and even panic. So, if you meet someone with autism and you feel strangely invisible, it may be because all they are able to focus on is that bit of fluff on your T-shirt, not you.

ASPERGER SYNDROME
What is it?
This is a neurological condition and is a high-functioning form of autism and an inability to interact socially (see also autistic-spectrum disorder above). These children, however, do not have delayed language or intelligence skills. Asperger symptoms will often be identifiable in obsessive interest in objects rather than toys, in rough play and avoidance of affection, and in clumsiness and resistance to change. From around five years old and upwards, these children will expect strict adherence to rules and will be unusually focused on gathering or collating objects or discussing them. They can be prone to extreme anxiety and to withdrawing from the world around them.

How yoga can help
Your goal is to develop a trusting bond with your child, observe what interests them in terms of postures and where their interests might lie. Try to integrate these interests as much as possible within the story. Yoga will help children to have a greater physical awareness of their body and how it moves, which may help to make them higher-functioning individuals in terms of age-appropriate goals. Often, children who are autistic and those who have Asperger benefit from the strengthening effects of the posture work. Very often these children have very low muscle tone and are extremely flexible. Yoga postures help to build strength around the vulnerable areas of the joints while helping to develop muscle tone. In addition, calming and tension-releasing exercises can be suitable for reducing coping mechanisms such as hand-flapping.

Praise your child for their postures, which will in turn help improve their self-esteem. Use descriptive praise such as 'I like the way you snap your arms in crocodile or stand so straight in tree' instead of just using, 'Good, well done' or empty praise, so that they know exactly what they have done well.

Children with Asperger also find it difficult to be anything other than themselves, so it is through trust and instruction that they become familiar with the postures. These children and those on the autistic spectrum suffer from 'overload'. This is when there is too much noise or activity or too many people around them. It is important to recognise when they need quiet time away from noise and interruption.

CEREBRAL PALSY
What is it?
This condition can manifest in three ways and affects the motor areas of the brain, i.e. the ability to control the muscles and body movement. On the whole, the condition develops during pregnancy or at childbirth through illnesses such as meningitis or through severe head injuries, which can cause the onset of the condition, although there can also be genetic reasons.

Some children will have a combination of symptoms, although possibly the most common form is spastic cerebral palsy, when the muscles, through overcontraction, are resistant to movement. They may have no cognitive or intellectual impairment at all.

Athetoid cerebral palsy will be characterised by involuntary movements such as writhing, drooling and twisting, due to their muscles changing rapidly from tense to floppy. There may also be hearing problems and speech difficulties.

Symptoms of ataxic cerebral palsy will affect balance and children find it difficult to remain upright without swaying due to spatial awareness difficulties.

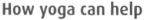

How yoga can help
Yoga is perfectly suited for most children with cerebral palsy, since it helps to reduce areas affected by high muscle tone so that the body is able to move more freely. This is achieved through stretching the muscles, and also through mobilising the spine, and in turn releasing pressure on the discs, which reduces muscular tension through the radial nerves. Also, due to issues with spatial awareness, they may present as clumsy.

The posture work not only helps to release tight muscles but also helps to strengthen weak muscles (low muscle tone) in other areas. Postural alignment works on both over- and underdeveloped muscle groups, because it is such a comprehensive way of exercising the body. Try to introduce postures at floor level if your child finds it difficult to balance.

It may well be necessary to manipulate the child's body for them, especially children who are wheelchair users – be careful to maintain the correct alignments, even in the limbs you are not working on.

In order to reduce high muscle tone in the calves, encourage the children to walk on their heels, which benefits them greatly.

DOWN'S SYNDROME
What is it?
Down's is a condition present from birth and is genetic. It is characterised by various physical characteristics, such as enlarged tongue and learning difficulties, and particular medical conditions, such as conductive hearing loss and visual impairments, including long- or short-sightedness and squints, heart conditions, higher-than-average susceptibility to colds and infections (particularly respiratory chest infections), and low muscle tone.

Children are normally shorter than average. Unfortunately, too, having a weaker immune system means they are more prone to illness but are extremely flexible and also generally affectionate.

How yoga can help
The function of the lymphatic system is improved through posture work, which in turn aids the immune system. These postures include chest thumping and knee hugging. Likewise, the endocrine system is strengthened, and this can help with stabilising weight, since children with Down's are more prone to weight gain. Seated forward bends are helpful in working on the endocrine system.
Some children with Down's syndrome have atlanto-axial instability (their top cervical vertebrae are weak). If you are not the parent,

do check with them beforehand to know whether this condition is present. If it is, the child should therefore avoid inverted postures with extreme flexion of the neck (such as the Fish pose) and other postures that might put pressure on their cervical vertebrae. Other inverted postures, such as downward Dog, do not pose a threat. Ensure that knees and elbows are slightly bent to prevent hypermobility.

SENSORY-INTEGRATION DYSFUNCTION
What is it?
The main task of our central nervous system is to integrate the senses, and over 80 per cent of our nervous system is involved in processing or organising sensory input, and thus the brain is primarily a sensory processing machine.

Sensory integration is a complex subject, since children with sensory-integration dysfunction may demonstrate one or more of the following characteristics:

* poor spatial awareness;
* difficulty in paying attention;
* poor response to stimulus;
* unco-ordinated body movements;
* inability to execute fine motor skills.

These indications may cause a child to feel lethargic or hyperactive and awkward.

There are generally two types of sensory integration dysfunction: overstimulated and understimulated. The overstimulated child will be the one who has more difficulty concentrating (the feeling they experience is like that of a child coming off a merry-go-round). The understimulated child would have difficulty concentrating because of their low arousal levels, and these children would benefit by integrating their senses such as by sitting on a wobbly cushion, chewing something or stroking a soft toy.

Our understanding of sensory integration is relatively new. It involves using the senses to improve concentration techniques. For example, a child who is stimulated only visually (such as by television) may benefit (as we noted) from sitting on a wobbly cushion or perhaps chewing something. This will help to balance and aid auditory function (hearing sense) and improve learning ability.

We operate through a combination of 'far' senses – smell, taste, seeing, hearing and touch. However, we also use the 'near' senses, which, to most of us are much less familiar. These are the vestibular sense of the inner ear, the tactile sense of the skin and the proprioceptive sense of the muscles and joints. The near senses are not ones we can control directly. They are responsible for the regulation of the internal organs, temperature, digestion, mood, etc.

The vestibular sense processes information about movement, gravity and balance via the inner ear. The tactile sense processes information via touch, mainly through the skin. The proprioceptive sense deals with information about body position and body parts, which is received through the muscles, ligaments and joints. The near senses are vital to a child's healthy development and their contact with the outside world.

How yoga can help

Yoga increases body and spatial awareness, while improving co-ordination, stamina and flexibility. It helps to teach a child serenity and strength in themselves, so that they are more able to manage their own challenges.

Many of the YogaBugs adventures include postures that benefit the sensory functions and indeed improve them with practice. Stroking and tapping, such as applying sun cream (see Page 24), adding the contents to our sandwich (Page 156) and being a Gorilla (Page 148) can help children with sensory dysfunction, while rocking (rocking and rolling, Page 133) and rotating postures (twists like Deer, Page 143) and Mermaid, Page 152) can help children with vestibular dysfunction. Standing postures are weight-bearing: Tree (Page 159), Surfer (Page 158) and Magic Bird (Page 152) can all send sensory information through the muscles and joints. Likewise, rolling has a squeezing effect (rock and rolling) on the muscles and joints.

These postures and movements can help children with proprioceptive dysfunction. In addition, postures that involve pushing (such as the Dog pose, see Page 143) can help the brain to get the correct feedback. It is interesting, too, to begin the session lying down, then moving slowly to all fours and then transferring to standing postures, since this reminds the brain of the developmental processes.

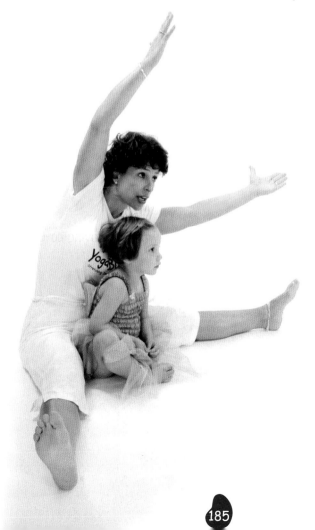

Appendix
How YogaBugs Came About

My journey into the world of yoga came as something of a surprise. I had no idea what a profound effect it would have on me, my family and my career and how its powerful influence would always be present thereafter in my daily life. Yoga has turned out to be a real soulmate.

I went on a 'walkabout' to India with my very good friend, Sarah Muirhead. We had met at a language school in the South of France when we were eighteen. Our friendship has continued and our shared interest in yoga has flourished. We were twenty-five when we started our practice on a beach in Kerala, southwest India. We had met a yoga teacher from Poland called Stefan, who had just completed his training with the world famous Mr Iyengar himself and was a motivated and enthusiastic teacher. We were captivated by his enthusiasm.

I remember being a little alarmed that my mother used to practise yoga when she was going through her leotard-and-brown-bread days, but, as a child, I was a gymnast, and now, years later, yoga seemed to embody a lot of what I had loved in terms of stretching, twisting and turning upside down and inside out! Stefan swiftly dispelled any preconceptions, and our daily classes were held overlooking the setting sun across the Indian Ocean.

When I returned to London a few months later, the best thing happened. I met Kay Fowler. Kay is unique, an inspired yogi, a magical person whose honesty and spirituality are true and beautiful, and I thank her for everything that has followed. Kay's Chelsea classes were packed, and everyone adored her. I was so inspired by her that I decided, after a few years of Kay's classes, that I wanted to train to become a yoga teacher myself. I signed up with the British Wheel of Yoga on their teacher-training course in London.

After India, I returned to the travel industry (my previous career) and was involved in organising overseas incentive trips for companies who wanted to develop the loyalty and commitment of their employees. Yoga fitted well into this life, because I was able practise it anywhere, and found to my surprise that the most unlikely people were taking to the yoga mat too. It is such a universal activity wherever you go or whatever your age.

I moved to work with an International Hotel Group and found myself taking conference and incentive organisers around the world to sample our different five-star hotel properties. While the job seemed glamorous and exciting, I felt that I wanted to be at home more and travel less. I had by this time met Rob, my husband-to-be, and, not surprisingly, travelling was the last thing on my mind!

Over time Rob and I started to practise together and he too got bitten by the yoga bug! When our individual jobs changed we decided it was time for something different and we were ready to explore new horizons. We both went on a yoga teacher-training course and returned to set up our own yoga and complementary-health centre which we called the Art of Health.

Writing now, I find it hard to believe that we have Felix (eleven), Barney (seven) and Letty (five) plus my stepson, George (sixteen) – and then there's Alfred, a bossy and very manly dachshund! George (who was our original YogaBug), now being a teenager, is busy investigating life ahead of him and exploring the new freedom that his age brings him. Felix is a sociable guy, very into fashion, sport and cool music. Barney is a thinker, a sensitive soul, artistic and deliciously loving. Letty is their squeezy and adorable little sister, determined to keep up with everything that her boys do!

My life is a constant juggling act between work deadlines, teaching yoga classes, taking the children to after-school activities all over southwest London, jogging three times a week, playing for a women's tennis team and having a busy social life with local friends. I could not do any of it without the support and understanding of Rob, the children, my fantastic parents, Lara Goodbody, my invaluable and tireless business partner, and those precious moments on the yoga mat.

I want to share with you the valuable connection that I have found through yoga with my family and friends. I would like children to explore yoga using our suggested stories and I would like you, the adult, to see the benefits. Whether your child jumps in feet first with you or holds back and just watches for a while, he or she will always gain some value from yoga, bringing a new dimension to creativity and movement.

I'll illustrate this with a true story. One of our YogaBugs teachers, Nisha, once told me of a child who arrived at her weekly class in school and wrapped herself up in her yoga mat to observe the class from under a table. Nisha was concerned that the child did not appear to want to take part, but was amazed to hear from her mother how much she adored her yoga classes. She told Nisha that every week her daughter would come home and take the entire family through the story. They would all be down on the floor following her every move and instruction!

WHAT HAPPENED NEXT

In 1997 our first YogaBugs were born. They grew out of the Art of Health and Yoga Centre in southwest London and there are now about forty thousand of them taking part in classes every week during term time. We have trained more than 1,200 teachers throughout the UK and Ireland, and there's growing interest in the US, Australia, Europe and Asia! The Art of Health closed in 2003 due to the relentless demand from property developers in the area. Perhaps it can be seen as fortuitous because, with hundreds of people visiting the centre each week, the building was being stretched to capacity!

YogaBugs was registered as a limited company in 2003. In December of the same year, Laura Harcourt, who had also been a director of the Art of Health, joined the team and Lara, who had been running her own business in Dublin, came on board as managing director. She subsequently married my brother Nick (they had met a few years previously). This was the best thing that could have happened for both our families, for YogaBugs and of course for them. Nick is our ideas man, full of ingenious thoughts and suggestions and powered by the expertise of a sizable London marketing company. He and Lara have recently produced their own little YogaBug, Richie, who will shortly be taking to his yoga mat!

One of our key goals over the next few years is to bring yoga for children to the attention of the government and to highlight the values for young children of all-inclusive and noncompetitive classes. Issues of obesity, low self-esteem, vulnerable immune systems, back problems and lack of exercise have all combined to make yoga a natural choice before, during and after the school day. We would like to give children a solid foundation in an activity that is not only a healthy exercise, but a valuable support to them for the rest of their lives.

The unique story-style approach of YogaBugs has generated huge interest from the media in the shape of newspapers, magazines and radio. TV coverage has included BBC2's *Dragon's Den*, GMTV, BBC2's *Working Lunch, This Morning* and *ITN News*.

YogaBugs is continuing to develop the teacher-training programme in the UK and expanding it as a franchise model for the UK and overseas. Naturally, this will combine to increase awareness about yoga and enable more children to practise at home and at school in many different countries around the world.

Here in the UK, YogaBugs sessions have been observed by inspectors from OFSTED (the UK schools regulating body). They have commented that the structure seems to integrate key aspects of children's learning, and yoga is particularly suited to the emotional, personal and social development of the child. All of this fits with the child's personal learning plan in terms of expressing appropriate feelings, needs and preferences and forming positive relationships with other children and adults.

We hope to see some happy and positive results from your own YogaBugs. Enjoy the book!

Acknowledgements

I would like to thank Kay Fowler, my inspiration in yoga who has been a true friend together with her husband Harry. Ursula Schoon-raad, for her wisdom through Iyengar Yoga, has always been a constant source of support to me. And my thanks to David Life and Sharon Gannon who have created the coolest yoga in the world through their Jivamukti classes!

I would also like to acknowledge the dedication and spirit of friend-ship from staff, teachers, therapists and clients in those years at The Art of Health and Yoga Centre. My gratitude as well to Suzy Cindrich, likeminded yogi Stateside, who provides a magical mixture of hu-mour and understanding.

I would like to thank my wonderful parents (Richard and Carol) for their tireless support and encouragement, my husband Rob for his love and all that he does to keep our life running happily and smoothly, my children, Felix, Barney and Letty and my stepson George. I couldn't have done any of this without my amazing sister in law, business partner and soul mate Lara Goodbody and the won-derful Emilie Despois who keeps us all on track. Finally, I would like to thank all my dear friends and yoga students for their enthusiastic belief in me.

Index